Praise for *The Little*

D1551455

"Carol Martin has created a one-stop sho
eminently readable and nicely walks you .
using personal experiences to educate and inform. Every patient
considering liposuction is well advised to read this book cover to cover."

—James Wells, MD, FACS, Long Beach, CA
Past President, American Society of Plastic Surgeons

"The Little Book of Lipo is a comprehensive guide that accurately
prepares patients for the experience they have when considering and
undergoing liposuction. Many of the anecdotes and suggestions could
easily be applied to just about any area of cosmetic surgery. Carol
Martin's experience as a patient and advisor allow her to give a very
accurate account of what to expect when contemplating liposuction."

—Jeffrey Kenkel, MD, FACS
Dallas, TX

"The Little Book of Lipo brings a treasure trove of practical guidance for
the patient considering liposuction. 'Is it right for me?' 'What are
reasonable expectations?' 'How do I know I've found the right surgeon?'
'How do I best prepare for surgery and recovery?' Carol Martin answers
all of these questions and many more in a clear and witty style. Follow
her advice and you will be well on your way to enjoying the wonderful
changes that liposuction can bring."

—Felmont F. Eaves III, MD, FACS
Charlotte, NC

"I have been in the arena of plastic surgery for 13 years. I have visited
many medical congresses, talked to many doctors, nurses, and even patients
that have had different types of surgery. After reading Carol Martin's book,
I can say only one thing: Where was this book before I had my own
liposuction? The book provides a wealth of accurate information. By
reading this book, patients will be much more prepared and informed about
their operations. The knowledge that comes from this book will ensure
better results and yield more value from the money they invest."

—Vera Watkins, Co-founder, The Marena Group
www.marenagroup.com (post-surgical compression garments)

Hope you enjoy the Book!
Carol

The Little Book of Lipo

Everything You Need to Know about Liposuction but Didn't Know to Ask!

Carol Martin

Busystreet Press

Carol Martin's Little Book of Lipo

Copyright ©2007 by Carol M. Martin

The companies and products whose names appear
in this book for purposes of example or
recommendation retain all rights of trademarks or
registered trademarks of their respective
company and product names.

ISBN 978-1-4196-6543-1

All rights reserved. No part of this book may be reproduced,
stored in a retrieval system, or transmitted, in any form or
by any means, without express written permission of the
publisher, Busystreet Press, 1579 Monroe Dr., Ste. F 922,
Atlanta, GA 30324.

This book is for informational purposes; the author provides no express or
implied warranty of any type and makes no representations about the
suitability of these materials for any purpose other than to provide
information. Neither The Informed Choice, Inc., nor Carol M. Martin shall
have any liability whatsoever for any use of this book.

Cover design by Shawn Spann and Rebecca Cashwell
of Quadras, Inc.

Cover photo by Rick Newby of Rick Newby Photography.

Text design and editing by Zuzana Urbanek, Z-ink.

*A percentage of all book sales will go to the
The Chelko Foundation.
www.thechelkofoundation.org*

First printing November 2007.
Printed in the United States of America.

www.theinformedchoice.com

Dedication

This book is dedicated to two people whose lives are benchmarks in the world I cover and call my own.

When **Dr. John Bostwick** died in 2001, we lost a great surgeon, and I lost a great friend. Back in the 1980s, I chose him to do my first liposuction. Not only did he have the credentials, he inspired amazing trust and confidence. As a surgeon and a human being, he just connected with his patients in a very special way, and he connected with me.

Later, when I explored starting my consultation business, I called him for an appointment to talk about some ideas. I arrived a few minutes early, but instead of putting me in an examining room, his secretary led me to his office. It wasn't large, but it was filled with books that he'd authored and photographs of family and friends—very warm, very cozy. As I stood there reading a plaques, he opened the door and greeted me with a big hug. "To what do I owe this honor?" he asked.

I blurted out my business idea, and he though it was great. He said I'd already referred more people than any other patient he'd ever had. I told him that was a no-brainer, when all I wanted was for others to feel as happy with their surgery as I was. (The breast augmentation he did for me has lasted 25 years without one problem.)

Suddenly, he turned to his books, grabbed several, and handed them to me. "Take these home and go through them," he told me. I returned them a few months later; I felt like I'd graduated from a mini-med school.

A few years later, I was in New York at a plastic surgery conference, where he was giving a speech about breast implants. As I walked towards the meeting room where he was speaking, the doors opened and hundreds of doctors poured out. I hoped to see him to say hello, but he was mobbed by a crowd of young doctors clamoring for his attention like fans of a rock star after a concert. When he saw me, he excused himself, walked over, and gave me a big hug. We caught up briefly, and I half-joked that he could trot me out as exhibit A—a satisfied patient. He laughed. But Dr. Bostwick also knew that WE knew he gave his patients more than a fine surgical fix; he gave us hope and a new outlook. We still talk and think about him. Dr. Bostwick set the bar.

Judy Loveless is someone I wish I'd met. While her story is tragic, her death may have saved other lives by giving surgeons a wake-up call. In 1997, Judy died from complications after surgery in a non-accredited outpatient clinic. I tell part of her story on pages 59–61 in this book.

Carol Martin's Little Book of Lipo
Acknowledgements

Special thanks (in no particular order) go to the following:

Sara Harris for the "little book" idea as well as all your help with this book!

Dr. Vincent Zubowicz for your patience and honesty.

Vera and Bill Watkins of The Marena Group, Dr. Christoper Patronella, Dr Monte Eaves, Dr. Mark Crispin, Dr. Diane Alexander, Dr. Jeff Kenkel, Dr. James Wells, Dr. James Baker, Dr. Brian Kinney, Dr. Laura Beaty, Dr. Mark Beaty, American Society for Aesthetic Plastic Surgery, Jill Sutton, Ford Smith for the fun cartoons, Ruby Mason for the wonderful drawings, David and Judy Russell, Comer Jennings, Stephen Camp, Mike Grandberry, Rick Newby, Danny Christensen, Joe Beck, Tillie Brush, Roger Smith, Rebecca Cashwell, and Shawn Spann.

All my buddies at *Atlanta Magazine*.

Dr. John G. Keating for giving me the idea to start my cosmetic surgery consulting business *The Informed Choice*.

Kathleen Askier.

All my clients whose brains I picked.

Helen and Cecil Alexander.

Randi Layne for always being there to hold my hand.

All my friends, too many to name…thanks for y'all's support through the years.

My parents, Ben and Mary Martin. Thank you for giving me the opportunity to do all the things any child could wish for.

My wonderful, sweet husband Art Harris for always believing in me.

Josh and Adam for always making me proud to be their step-mother.

AND the most important thanks of all—

Zuzana,

I could not have done this without my colleague and collaborator, Zuzana Urbanek, who has provided the magic words, the research, encouragement, and enthusiasm for this project, pulling out answers to questions I never knew I had inside, working thousands of hours on and off for seven years to help me shape and finish a book I'd only dreamed about doing, who inspired me when I hit the wall of doubt, who reminded me how much it could help others who feel—like I once did—overwhelmed and afraid as they wonder if they should have surgery or not—to offer reliable advice that will allow them to make an informed choice…and a safe one.

Carol Martin's Little Book of Lipo

Carol Martin's Little Book of Lipo

Table of Contents

Carol Martin's Little Book of Lipo

Foreword

Vincent N. Zubowicz, MD, FACS, Atlanta, GA
Owner and operator of CPS (Center for Plastic Surgery)

I can only pity the consumer interested in getting rid of a little unwanted fat. In spite of the development of safe and reliable techniques, confusion reigns over the land of unwanted bulges and bags. There is a lot of money being spent and almost no regulation of aesthetic manipulations of the body. As a consequence, the market is full of carnival barkers and snake-oil salesman. There are so many techniques that are cheaper, safer, revolutionary, blah, blah, blah.

The consumer indeed needs an advocate, someone to sort through the rubbish and unveil the facts. Carol Martin does this magnificently in her "little" book on liposuction. It's very readable and based on detailed research and interviews with doctors who really know what works and what doesn't. You can trust what you learn from this book. There is no agenda here except to educate the consumer. You won't find this kind of unbiased information in the Yellow Pages or on someone's Web site.

Liposuction, with all its variations, has been around for many years and has an enviable record when examining specialists with proper training. *In properly selected patients* the results are predictably good. The operation is amazingly safe with very few complications, very small incisions, and brief convalescence.

Because there is profit without oversight, many declare themselves practitioners and market their services to the unsuspecting public. Fortunately they are in the minority, but they seem to be the ones that make the most noise. Carol gives you the tools to sort them out. If you are the right patient and find your way to a competent doctor, you will love what liposuction can do.

Read the book. Understand the techniques and alternatives. Keep your expectations realistic. Ask the right questions. Seek out a good doctor. It's all in the forthcoming pages.

Why should you read this book?

I want you to go into cosmetic surgery with your eyes open!

Well, not literally. You'll probably want to be sedated.

What I mean is, you need to be realistic and understand what lies ahead. When it comes to cosmetic surgery (also known as plastic surgery), you need to have information about the latest techniques and about what surgery can do—and what it *cannot*. Many people go into surgery without a realistic understanding of the physical facts behind the procedure they are about to have done. And even more people think they will turn back the hands of time in a radical way by having a facelift or tummy tuck. Don't let fantasies mix with the facts when it comes to something as important as your health and safety—be aware and make a knowledgeable choice.

You need to know how **to prepare for your procedure**, preparing not only yourself but also your family and others in your life, as well as your home and routine. I will walk you through step-by-step plans for everything from what to eat (and not eat) before surgery, to making arrangements for a successful recovery.

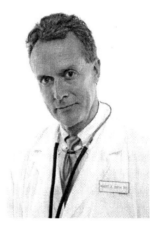

Without question, the most important thing you need to know is **how to find the best surgeon**. How do you assess that he is the best for you? The best ways are not through his advertising or his reputation around town as a good golfer or

3

well-known supporter of the arts. And where do you get the real scoop about where he studied, his credentials, and what experience he has in his practice?

(Excuse me for using only the male pronoun when referring to doctors, but the fact is that the majority of cosmetic surgeons today are male, though the number of female surgeons is growing, and let's face it...it's easier than saying "he or she" all the time! By the time this book hits its second edition, perhaps we'll see a shift, and I'll have to use that awkward he/she combination thing!

Answering questions about preparation, recovery, finding the right surgeon, and many other questions, is where I come in. I'm not a doctor, and I won't be giving you any medical advice in this book (except to pass along advice from doctors themselves), but I have earned the confidence and trust of cosmetic surgeons. The good ones are as concerned about the well-being and satisfaction of their patients (as well as the reputation and success of cosmetic surgery) as I am. They talk to each other, and they talk to me. Like a reporter who covers a field, my "beat" is cosmetic surgery, the doctors who perform it, and the people who choose to have it. What I have learned over the years, and continue to find out from doctors and their patients, allows me to help people choose their surgeon wisely and to make *informed* choices. It's why I named my consulting business **The Informed Choice**, and you need to know what I know if you are considering cosmetic surgery.

Some people who hear about my service seek me out as a last resort, after having poorly done procedures that their doctors won't or can't fix. I can usually help them find the right surgeon who is able to help. But it means more surgery, more recovery time, more pain, and more money. I don't want to be in the business of helping people get "fixed" after poorly done operations!

I want everyone who has cosmetic surgery to have a positive and rewarding experience and wind up with what they wanted to gain from it. One of the reasons I wrote this book is to reach more people with the "ounce of prevention" before they to need to seek me out for such distressing cures.

Let's face it, a great many things in life are not in our control: even the best doctor can have a bad day; surgery always carries risks of problems and complications; our own bodies may sometimes choose to react differently to being invaded than we or our doctors expect. But it is *not* luck—and don't let anyone tell you it is.

By being informed, you can anticipate and eliminate as many of the wild cards as possible. Minimize the risks by knowing what they are. Avoid the pitfalls that sometimes result in an unsatisfactory procedure.

It all sounds a bit scary, I know. The truth is, great results and happy patients are the rule—not the exception—in cosmetic surgery. But even if you're one in a million, *you* don't want to be the one to have the unfortunate problem!

Having cosmetic surgery is one of the most important decisions you will ever make in your life. It's right up there with decisions to get married, have a child, or buy a new house. And it's a lot more permanent than at least one of the three (the house...what did you think I meant?!).

Think about it: You'll actually be changing a part of your own body, the one you see every time you look in the mirror. Pretty big stuff. Amazingly, most people spend more time picking out a dress for an important party or coordinating their stereo equipment than they do scrutinizing which doctor is best qualified to perform their cosmetic surgery! There is a great deal people don't think about.

Did you know that

- any doctor with a medical license can perform cosmetic surgery?

- it is very difficult to sue a cosmetic surgeon if you are unhappy with the results of your procedure?

- quoted fees may not include pre-op lab work, the operating room, anesthesia, and other hidden costs?

- it can take up to a year to heal fully?

It's your body. You should be in charge. To be in control of your decision, you need to be armed with the facts.

This book is a comprehensive, no-nonsense guide for anyone considering liposuction or a procedure in which it is used. In these pages, you'll find your fears addressed, you'll read information about liposuction, you'll read about others who have had a variety of experiences, and you'll receive step-by-step advice for making sure you get the best results possible.

Why I wrote this book

In over 20 years of research into cosmetic surgery, a dozen personal cosmetic procedures, and assisting hundreds of others as a patient advocate and consultant, I have never come across a book that offers what I long to provide my clients—a simple and visual "tell all" manual that helps people become informed patients.

So I decided to write it myself!

In 1990, I was a model and actor living in Atlanta, Georgia. (Yes, I'm a Southern girl, born in Georgia and still living in Atlanta today.) I had had three cosmetic procedures and knew many people—male and female—in the entertainment industry that used cosmetic surgery as one way to keep the looks that put bread on the table.

I was fascinated with cosmetic surgery, and being around a lot of people who had the occasional "nip and tuck"—even before it became so popular—fueled my interest. It also allowed me to explore what other people went through, adding their experiences to my own.

That year, 1990, I appeared on the cover of *Atlanta* magazine for a feature on cosmetic surgery. I didn't know it at the time, but apparently so many people were starved for information about it, this issue became the biggest seller of the year and among the top ten best-selling issues in the history of the publication.

After the issue hit the stands, I was contacted by dozens of people seeking information about doctors, procedures, and what to expect with cosmetic surgery. It concerned me that so many of the callers were willing to pay huge sums for cosmetic surgery when they didn't have a realistic understanding of the procedure they wanted to have and didn't know what to look for in a doctor's credentials. I realized there was a real need for solid information about cosmetic surgery.

Before my own operations, I had always set realistic expectations, conducted thorough research about the procedure I would be having, and interviewed several surgeons. I also prepared for the procedure, and I followed my doctor's instructions during recovery. Most people, I found out, did not know some or all of these steps to getting the best results. I decided to offer my experience to others.

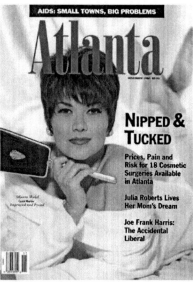

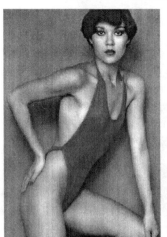 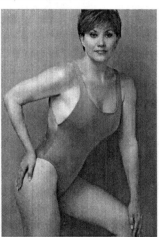

The cover of Atlanta *magazine that started it all (top).*
Carol at age 22(bottom left) and at age 50 (right).

In 1995, I founded **The Informed Choice**, a consulting service for people interested in having cosmetic surgery. The Informed Choice was the first cosmetic surgery information and referral service in the nation. While others now offer similar services, The Informed Choice remains dedicated to meeting clients' needs. We provide up-to-date information about procedures, physicians' credentials and experience, referrals to qualified doctors, ways to prepare for the operation, how to make recovery as smooth as possible, referrals for recovery care, recommendations about helpful products, and much more. Most importantly, we give people the peace of mind that comes with knowing they are informed and in control of the major decision they are making about their bodies.

Today, I am recognized as a national expert on cosmetic surgery, with credits such as Entertainment Tonight, CNN, the Fox Network, and *Glamour*, to name a few. My mission is simple: to utilize my years of experience to guide people through lengthy and confusing surgical information, assist them in finding the most qualified surgeon, and help them make an informed choice to achieve the great results they deserve. I'm serious about what I do, and I bring a wealth of solid research to every recommendation I make. I also love my job. I feel fortunate each and every day that I can apply my experiences to helping others. I am there for my clients to turn to with questions and for guidance. With this book, I want to assist, educate, and bring peace of mind to an even greater number of people.

I applaud those people who want to grow old gracefully. More power to you! But I am not one of that group. I am in that camp of people who use everything at our disposal—nutrition, exercise, rest, skin care, AND cosmetic surgery—to become what we want to be and to stay that way. Nobody is the perfect size or shape, nobody is symmetrical, and nobody stays young-looking forever.

Cosmetic surgery is not an exact science, but it can help us to get closer to looking on the outside the way we feel inside.

Enjoy reading this book. More importantly, let it serve as a guidebook in becoming informed about the choice you make to have cosmetic surgery. Use it as a reference and focus on what you have questions about. Or, read it from cover to cover. If you do read it all the way through, you'll find some points repeated a few times. Take note—it means they're important; remember when your mother said, "If I have to tell you one more time..."? Often the little point can make a world of difference. It never hurts to hear important things one more time!

An informed patient is the best patient!

Carol M. Martin

Carol M. Martin

To have or not to have... liposuction

That's the question you need to ask yourself first.

For some people, making the decision is the toughest part. Do you really need to have something done? Are you doing for it for yourself or because of pressure from someone else? After all has been said and done, will it be worth it for you?

Make a list

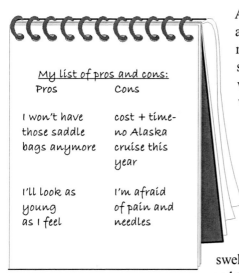

My list of pros and cons:

Pros

I won't have those saddle bags anymore

I'll look as young as I feel

Cons

cost + time- no Alaska cruise this year

I'm afraid of pain and needles

A list is something I ask all my clients to make. On the positive side, you may write what cosmetic surgery will allow you to change...something that bothers you, like the love handles that hours of aerobics won't shrink. On the not-so-positive side, there is the cost, pain, bruising, swelling, possible risks, and time to recover.

Are you thinking that cosmetic surgery will change your life? Well, it can. But it can't give you a new one. Look at all the ugly ducklings with, say, a big nose and no chin, who turn into bombshells on *Extreme Makeover* or *The Swan*. Whether you like the shows or not, you have to admit they've transformed many men and women physically, and many report that the boost in self-esteem and self-confidence DOES change their lives in a positive way. After all, we are all judged by our appearance, like it or not—I didn't make that rule. And liposuctioning those saddle bags that you've always wanted to get rid of might give you just the boost you need.

In most cases, the results can be very good, but they *may not* live up to the fantasies we carry around deep inside. It's going to take a lot of hard work on your part, plus a very skilled surgeon, to go from double-chinned roly-poly to supermodel, and that enormous transformation may never happen.

Also, we all carry psychological baggage that can undermine any program of self improvement. Unless we unpack it along the way and air it out and understand why we got how we are, we could wind up in the same pickle again, no matter how great we may look. I don't want my clients to set themselves up for disappointment. They will be the same people as before, I tell them, only better-looking. So, the list is done to help understand themselves and their motivations better.

Why do *you* want to have liposuction?

Here are some questions to ask yourself when figuring out why exactly you want to have liposuction. Of course, you need to consider your own needs and motivations much more carefully and in detail, but these can get you started. How many of these statements do you say "yes" to? Some are legitimate motivations to consider cosmetic surgery. But some are warning signs that you may need something other than a cosmetic procedure.

1. Doing aerobics six times a week still doesn't take the bulges off some places.

   Bulges that simply will not go away with proper diet and exercise can be removed through procedures such as liposuction or a tummy tuck.

2. Your friend has had liposuction and is getting all the attention. And you're not.

   I categorically advise you against having cosmetic surgery to "keep up" with anyone. This isn't a new car or a party dress you're buying—it's surgery! We all react differently to the trauma of an operation, so you may not have the same results as the person you're envying. A good rule of thumb is to consider that, if no one else were around, would you still want to change what you're thinking of changing. In other words, are you doing it for yourself? If not, then don't do it!

3. When you look in the mirror, you're reminded of a centerfold—unfortunately not a *Playboy* centerfold but more like something out of *National Geographic*!

   If gravity has taken over despite healthy eating and regular exercise, several cosmetic surgery procedures can help you regain a more youthful figure. They include such procedures as a breast lift, tummy tuck, and body lift, all of which usually include liposuction.

4. Friends look at you and ask when the baby is due.

If you have some unusually bulgy areas that really bother you—like a protruding stomach or saddlebags—liposuction can be the answer that dieting and exercise may never be.

5. Your significant other left you for someone younger, and you're thinking, "I've got shoes older than she is!"

   Never consider having surgery after an emotionally traumatic event, such as the break-up of a relationship or loss of job or a loved one. I highly recommend waiting a year after a dramatic life change before considering cosmetic surgery. Above all, don't think that having an operation will change anything that's happened.

Why people have cosmetic surgery

There are perfectly legitimate reasons for people to have cosmetic surgery, including liposuction. Granted, cosmetic procedures are elective, meaning they are operations one does not need to have to stay healthy or alive. Cosmetic surgery is a way to look younger and to fix what we see as imperfections, just like make-up, hairstyling, and flattering clothing.

The people with the most successful results are those who go into the procedure with realistic expectations and positive thoughts, choose a terrific surgeon, and then follow the doctor's recommendations to the letter.

I have also heard a few of my clients say that, all of their lives, they had done things for others. When they decided to have cosmetic surgery, it was the ultimate gift just for themselves.

Essential reasons NOT to have liposuction

There are some reasons that should make you stop and think twice, if not change your mind altogether, about wanting to have liposuction.

- First and foremost—and I know I'm repeating this, but it's that important—don't think that having liposuction will change your life completely! (It can, however, greatly boost your self-esteem.)

- Don't have liposuction to exact revenge—it won't affect anyone but you.

- Don't have it because you're jealous. You'll just add physical healing time and expense to your list of frustrations.

- Don't have it because you're depressed. Seek professional counseling!

- Don't do it because your significant other says you need it. It's your body, and it's up to you to decide. (Florida surgeon Dr. James Baker says it well: "I would not do implants if it's for a boyfriend or a husband who wants them. I would say to bring him in and we'll augment him! If he wants breasts, we'll put them in him.")

- Don't have it to make yourself "perfect." This is not an exact science, and if you think you'll look exactly like the movie star whose hips or flat stomach you want, you're setting yourself up for disappointment. You won't be satisfied.

Dr. Jeffrey Kenkel of Dallas, Texas, reminds patients that it is truly up to them to do what's needed to have the body they want. "I tell patients that surgery only gets you 50 to 60 percent there...the rest is up to the patient."

There are also some practical considerations. You may want to have liposuction for all the right reasons, but if you can't be an involved and responsible patient, it may not make sense, at least at present. For example, don't have a procedure if you can't take enough time off to recover. This includes reasons like having a demanding job, young children, and other responsibilities that you can't be away from or that are physically strenuous. Also, don't decide to have it right before a big event, like a class reunion or wedding. Depending on how extensive the liposuction is that you're having, you might be a bit swollen or bruised, or you may have complications (rare, but they do happen) and not be able to attend at all! And please consider finances carefully, and don't have it if it will drain you or put you in financial jeopardy. All this is to say, don't take having this procedure lightly!

What do you want your results to be?

Is it really liposuction you need, or a diet and exercise? Well, you may need both. Many people see cosmetic surgery as a quick fix for flab and extra weight. It really should be the last resort for stubborn problems that nothing else will alleviate.

Whatever the procedure you are considering, read up on it and understand the typical results it produces. Believe what you read and what doctors you interview tell you! When the literature and doctors tell you that you have a higher chance of loose skin after lipo, believe them!

Liposuction can, however, be one of many ways to improve some bothersome feature or get closer to an ideal of the most attractive you that you can be. And there's a lot to be said for that.

How do you make the final decision?

With everything there is to consider, you may wonder how you'll ever be sure. Well, some people are certain that liposuction is what they want. If you're one of them, congratulations! But please still do your homework and include some of the things you read here that you may not have thought about. If you're not that sure yet, here's a quick list that might make it easier.

- First, it needs to be your decision and yours alone. Certainly, get advice from those you trust, read, see a consultant if you wish. In the end, make the decision on your own. You—and you alone—will live with the results for a long time.

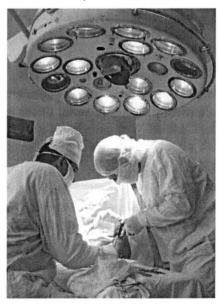

- Make sure the change you're looking for is one *you* want for *yourself.*

- If the thought of going under the knife absolutely terrifies you, or you have a negative attitude about what might happen (for example, all you think about are the risks), then don't do it. If you think it will go badly, it very well might. A positive attitude goes a long way!

- Some people think they need lots of work, and they're scared to do it all at once. If you're one of them, do it in phases and at your own pace. Get a little lipo, see how it goes, and perhaps a year later, get that tummy tuck you also want.

- If you have a family you take care of, you'll need to spend time away from them. You'll need to focus on yourself during recovery. Make sure you factor this into your decision.

- If you are at high risk for any type of surgery, consider whether it is worth that risk. If you see enough doctors, someone is bound to say they will do it for you despite the risks. Be honest with yourself—if four out of five surgeons you see recommend against it, do you really want to defy that?

It's OK if you decide to wait. Think about whether you really want to have liposuction. If you are not sure for any reason that it's exactly what you want, this is not the right time to do it. Just hold off. You can always do it later, when you are positive it's what you want. Believe me, the doctors will still be around!

When you do go forward, that's when the real work starts. That's when you'll really need to prepare yourself, your home, your loved ones, your work place, your finances, and more. So keep reading. In the coming chapters, I'll tell you all about how to get ready for what's ahead.

So, you want to have liposuction. Now what?

If you're reading this chapter, then you have done your homework, read the introduction and first chapter, and made the decision to indeed have liposuction.

Congratulations!

Now, it's time to really get down to business. As you embark on having your procedure done, the key is to **plan, plan, and plan some more**. I hope you're reading this well before you have the liposuction you want!

Your surgeon is the key

The most important thing is to **find the best-qualified surgeon** to perform your operation. All the steps to do it right are in the chapter about doctors.

Plan for a successful recovery

A very important aspect is to **plan sufficient time to recover**. Cosmetic surgery is just that—surgery. Your body goes through trauma during liposuction. Don't underestimate the time healing takes. Yes, everyone is different, and we each heal at our own pace, but if you're thinking that you will be the exception and recover much faster than others, you're headed for possible disappointment. Don't even go there!

Your surgeon will give you more details and will make personalized recommendations about what you should and shouldn't do during recovery. **Follow the doctor's advice to the letter!**

As a rule, remember what recovery is for—**rest, recuperation, and quiet time**. Just because you know you'll have time off from work doesn't mean you should combine that time with anything strenuous you've wanted to catch up on, like painting the house or cleaning out the garage. Trust me, you will not feel well enough to take on projects anyway.

Counting your pennies

Part of thorough planning is to have the resources you need to make your operation and recovery as painless as possible, in every way. As you're thinking about the time you'll need off from work, make sure you consider how that may affect you financially. Some people are salaried and have vacation time saved up, so this won't necessarily apply. Others are independently wealthy and don't need to work in the first place, so it certainly doesn't apply. But many of us are in business for ourselves or in jobs, like sales, where today's work equals tomorrow's money. Have you saved enough not only for the operation but to see you through the time you won't be working during recovery?

After some procedures, you may not be able to do much for a while. Housework and anything involving lifting (even grocery

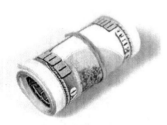
shopping) may not be options after some procedures. Because of this, there may be an **added cost to hire someone to do things** for you. Don't forget costs like childcare, pet boarding, transportation, and goods and

services delivered to your home when you can't go out.

The main financial considerations are, of course, the **costs of surgery**. I say "costs" because one has to consider a number of items besides the doctor's fee. Some of these include the operating room fee, anesthesia, medications, compression garments, and even possible home nursing care during recovery.

Throughout the time I have been a consultant, people have often asked about **how to get the money to have a cosmetic procedure** done, as the vast majority of these procedures are not covered by medical insurance. Here are some ideas:

- **Save up.** Have a separate account where you put your surgery savings, and have a plan for saving that you stick to.

- Get a **part-time job** to make extra money and save up faster. Even babysitting a few times each month can add up. Try tutoring, gardening for others, selling Tupperware or Mary Kay or Avon, working a few nights at a restaurant, or doing part-time office work. Be creative!

- Put the operation on a **credit card**. Most doctors today take credit cards; however, the anesthesiologist and operating room may not. If you have a credit card that offers cash advance checks, you can write one of these and no one will even know it's going on your credit card (but be aware that there is usually a fee from the card company for this).

- **Get a loan.** I have known several people who have taken out second mortgages of around $15,000 to cover all the costs of an operation like a tummy tuck. You don't have to say what it's for, and the interest rate is much cheaper than using a credit card. Plus, the interest may be tax deductible.

- Have the surgery **financed through the doctor's office** (many offer third-party financing nowadays) or an outside financing company that the office can recommend. Be aware that if you don't have good credit, you won't get the operation financed any more than you would a new car.

- Put your procedure on **"lay-away."** This is a very unusual method, and many doctors may not even consider it, but it's not a bad idea.

Several years ago, one of my clients told me how she was going to pay for her surgery. She made enough money to save for it, but she knew that if she put it aside somewhere that she had access to, she would dip into it. So she made an agreement with her doctor to pay him a certain amount per month until the procedure was paid in full. Then she had her operation. It's an ingenious idea, and if your surgeon agrees to it, you may find it a great way to go.

A few cautions, though: make sure you and the doctor have a written agreement outlining what happens to the money in the event the surgery cannot be performed for any reason (such as, you become ill or cannot have the operation for some reason, he closes his practice or moves to another state, or either of you passes away).

Little White Lies

Eight out of ten of my clients who have cosmetic surgery do not want others to know they've had it. If you're secretive about it, you're not alone. And it's OK to feel that way. It's no one else's business. So what do you 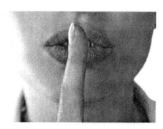 say when you don't want to admit, "I'm having liposuction"? Well, here are my "Little White Lies," which help you **prepare what you'll tell people** about why you'll be out of work or unable to do certain things during recovery.

Above all, **keep it simple**. Explain briefly, and don't embellish.

If you're having liposuction anywhere on your body:

- (Women) Say you're having some kind of female surgery—people are unlikely to ask further questions. Nosy people may pry further, so you may need to resort to that you just don't want to talk about it.

- (Men or women) Say you have a slipped disk in your back, or a pulled back muscle, or need a hernia repaired. These are good explanations for why you won't be able to lift or otherwise exert yourself for a while.

- Say you'll have a growth or cyst or mole removed. This works well to explain a small scar, as you would have from small-area liposuction.

Be careful—if you say you're having some other type of surgery, and you happen to be speaking with someone who may be interested in a referral to that type of doctor, make sure you have a name ready when they ask, "Oh, which doctor is doing that for you?"

People you won't be able to fool:

- It stands to reason that another doctor who examines you (like your family physician or your gynecologist), especially one who sees the area where you've had liposuction, will probably know what you had done. You also probably won't slip body surgery by a personal trainer, if you have one. You really should be honest with these people anyway, as they need to know for your own well-being and safety.

- If you have lipo of the cheeks, chin, or neck, you won't be able to hide it from people like your hairdresser or your dentist or your esthetician. Stress to them that you'd like to keep it confidential. If your hairdresser is the gossipy type, you may want to think about switching prior to having surgery. And with your dentist, it's important to talk about any facial surgery affecting the mouth or muscles in the lower face, for your own safety; if you know you need some dental work, it's best to schedule it before your cosmetic surgery, or at least six weeks after.

- Your spouse or significant other also should know.

There's something else to keep in mind. Have you ever had a friend who wore glasses for years, then got contact lenses, and you couldn't figure out why he or she looked different? Or a person (hopefully a man!) with a longtime mustache who shaved it off, and people puzzled over whether he'd lost weight? Have you had a zit on the end of your nose that you could swear announced your coming into the room like a neon sign, and when you pointed it out, no one else had noticed?

The changes you go through with liposuction will really be much more noticeable to you than to anyone around you. That's not to say a friend won't guess exactly what you had done. But I assure you that most people will not be preoccupied with finding out your secret, if you want to keep it as one.

Stop raining on my parade!

Criticism…horror stories…reasons you're not making the right choice…

There will always be someone ready to tell you you're doing the wrong thing. Often, it can be the person you least expect, like a sibling or a best friend. The more open you are about discussing your procedure, the more you can expect to hear. It's best to be prepared to handle these remarks.

People may be critical or negative for a number of reasons. People who care about you may not want you to change. Have you ever had someone who really does care about you seem to undermine efforts like dieting or getting a new hairstyle? It's as though they want you to fail at something that's good for you! I don't pretend to be a psychologist, but I know that there's something in many people that wants to keep those close to them just as they know them, warts and all.

Others may try to thwart your plans for other reasons. Perhaps they can't afford cosmetic surgery, so somehow they feel you shouldn't be able to have it either. They may secretly want to have it but are chicken (only the brave do it!). They may be jealous, and often will be even more so after your successful operation. Or they may simply not know enough about it and be frightened of cosmetic surgery as a concept. Seldom do people have well-supported reasons why cosmetic surgery should not be an option for you to pursue.

You can stop negative people in their tracks when you know what you're talking about. Being **armed with facts** gives you a big leg up. Usually they are relying on one story they heard or read about cosmetic surgery, and you will have a big advantage once you've done your homework.

Above all, remember to **stay grounded**. You are doing this for yourself. We all do things physically to make ourselves look and feel better. It's your body. You don't have to defend or explain yourself to anyone. If all else fails, tell people that if they can't be supportive, they should just leave it alone. It's no use getting into an argument.

If you can't think of clever comebacks for naysayers, it's OK. But just in case you'd like to have some retorts up your sleeve, here are examples of what to say in response to some ways people can put you through the mill:

Typical remark	Comeback
I saw this person on *20/20* who had cosmetic surgery and died!	What did this person know about his or her surgeon? (The fact is, people *very* rarely die from cosmetic surgery; hundreds of thousands who have undergone procedures are alive and happy!)
I can't believe you'd do something like that!	*Oh, I didn't realize I needed your approval! (jokingly) But if you'd like to hear about it, I'll tell you why I decided to do it.*

You look fine just as you are—you certainly don't need cosmetic surgery! (note: these are usually the same people who cross the room to whisper, "It's about time she did something about that!")

I appreciate you saying that, but I disagree. It's something I really want to do for myself.

Why would you change what God gave you?

God also gave us cosmetic surgeons. And God gave us flowers and bushes, and pruning enhances their beauty!

Couldn't you find something better to spend your money on?

I think the best thing I could spend my money on is myself!

Instead of liposuction, why don't you just exercise and diet?

Thanks for the suggestion, but I've been that route, and this is a problem it won't fix. (It's none of your beeswax anyway!)

"Am I being vain?"

We all judge others by appearance. For better or worse. Those are the rules, and I didn't make them up. What each of us needs to decide is how important others' judgments are to us, what we are happy with seeing in ourselves, and what we want to change that we're not happy with. Vanity? Well, yes, it's vain in a sense to put on make-up and nice clothes, to live in a beautiful home or drive an expensive car, and it's vain to have cosmetic surgery.

There are two kinds of vanity: positive vanity that makes us feel better about ourselves and hurts no one else, and negative vanity that obscures other values and allows a person to hurt others in pursuit of what he or she wants. As a cosmetic surgeon once told me, "bad vanity" is pathological preoccupation with appearance, while "good vanity" is self-critical personal evaluation with the desire to make positive changes for yourself, fully understanding the implications.

Let's talk about both.

We make ourselves look and feel better by wearing make-up, styling our hair, and putting on jewelry and flattering clothes. We can also eat right and exercise to produce more permanent change. Like all these other methods, cosmetic surgery is a way to change things we feel are flawed or imperfect. But you don't hear anyone saying, "You should be ashamed for whitening your teeth!" or "How vain of you to work out so much and spend your money on a personal trainer!"

I remember when I got my breasts. I was beside myself! For the first time in my life, I wasn't flat! It's a great feeling to put on a bathing suit or cocktail dress and feel really sexy (and know I look it!). There is nothing wrong with basking in that feeling! (But ladies, be careful—more men will inevitably look at you, and a boyfriend or husband can get very jealous. He'll need reassurance!)

Vanity begins to hurt us and others when we put the things that make us look and feel better before important and necessary values that should come first. A friend of mine has a sister who is dying to have a facelift. She found out how much it cost and realized she did not have that much expendable income, nor had she saved for it. Then it dawned on her that she really did have the money—in the savings she had put aside for her children's education.

Hold it! What's wrong with this picture?

Just as it would be wrong to buy a Mercedes with the education funds, it is wrong to use it for another unneeded expense like cosmetic surgery when the vital issue of the children's education is at stake. Likewise, it is possible to hurt ourselves unwisely, like using money set aside for rent and bills to pay for cosmetic surgery.

But let's say you've set aside disposable income for the operation you want, and your particular vanity will hurt no one. So what do you do when people try to make cosmetic surgery the worst of all evil vanities? To illustrate, let me tell you a story.

Have you ever had one of those wonderful experiences when you told someone to his or her face exactly what you thought and were able to back it up in an indisputable way? Rita (not her real name), a friend of a friend, once approached me at a dinner party, knowing I am a cosmetic surgery consultant.

"Heavy eyelids have always run in my family," she told me. "I can see mine starting to droop, but I'd never do anything about it. It's just so *vain*."

I looked at her and sized her up in about two seconds.

"Tell me, Rita, do you color your hair?"

"Why, yes."

"And back in school, did you wear braces on your teeth?"

"Yes."

"And your new car, didn't you say it was a Jag?"

"Yes, it is."

There you have it. It's really all vanity. Nobody *needs* a Rolex watch, or a Lexus, or a million-dollar mansion. Nobody *needs* to have longer lashes or fuller hair. And nobody *needs* cosmetic surgery. These are all things we choose to make ourselves look and feel good.

Oh, and by the way, Rita had her eyes done in 2005! She conveniently forgot what she said to me years ago.

As the story illustrates, you've got to be quick on your feet. If you know people or can quickly size up what their particular vanities are, ask them to tell you how that's different from yours, as I did in the story above. If you can't do that, or if they continue to argue with you, just ask, "How does my vanity hurt you? Why do you care so much that I'm doing this?"

Sometimes you'll encounter the true Earth Mother or Earth Father, a person natural to the core who doesn't see why someone would want to change themselves. You can't argue this one. Your belief systems are very different. Just tell them you admire them. "I'm impressed you're growing older gracefully. You seem happy, and you'll certainly save money! But I'm not like you."

There are also those people at the extreme of just not interested in taking care of themselves, often arguing that appearance does not matter at all. This is an argument called *reductio ad absurdum*, which basically means taking an argument to absurdity. The fact is, for better or worse, appearances DO matter. How you choose to deal with that fact is completely up to you.

Above all, it's important to always keep in mind that you are having your cosmetic surgery for yourself and no one else. As I said, if all else fails, ask people to just mind their own business!

Great expectations

We're not perfect going in, and we won't be perfect coming out. If you can remember this mantra, you'll be fine.

It is exceedingly important to go into liposuction with realistic expectations. **You will not be a different person.** Period. You will look better, and you'll feel better as a result of that. But please, please, please don't think—even in the back of your mind—that after lipo you will miraculously have a new life, save a failing relationship, or receive a long-overdue promotion. If you harbor any of these fantasies, you're setting yourself up for deep disappointment.

Cosmetic surgery is not a perfect science. You are made of flesh, muscle, and bone, which may react in unpredictable ways to the trauma of being surgically manipulated. **Things don't always turn out exactly as you and your surgeon planned**. Sometimes people have to have touch-ups. Know that this is a possibility.

Also, you need to have a realistic outlook about how long the healing process will take. It takes time and you'll need to **muster all your patience**. Your surgeon will give you an estimate of how long it will take you to heal (but he'll probably make the whole thing sound much easier than it is). This book also has some ranges. Prepare yourself psychologically for the healing to take the longest estimated time. That way, you will be pleasantly surprised when it doesn't take as long as you expected.

Part of the healing process is not expecting to look great for some time after the operation. Due to **swelling and bruising**, you will actually look worse at first! The swelling may be around for a while (although I've seen instances where it subsided quickly), so prepare yourself for that. You may even weigh more for a while (water weight). But it **will** eventually go down. It may take months, but it will get better all the time. Swelling and bruising will be worse some days and better others, and it may be worse (or better) for you than it was for someone else you know who had the same operation. People heal at different rates, so don't base your plans on someone else telling you it did not take as long. (Remember, too, that we tend to forget later how long things took.)

There are certainly some positive expectations you can have. One is that your **self-esteem will rise!** You're having something fixed that's been bothering you, so you'll look better in your own eyes and that will help you feel better about yourself. This will cause a boost in **confidence and comfort**, and you'll feel like you can take on the world! (Recall what it feels like to walk out of the hairdresser's with a killer new haircut—you feel like you could be a supermodel.)

One forewarning: if you always shied away from compliments before surgery, don't expect people to suddenly begin giving them after surgery. I spoke with a woman who was adamant that no one know about her facelift, then was disappointed that no one said she looked great. She had always been insecure and avoided compliments, so people knew not to give them anymore.

When it's new, what to do

Something to be very careful about in terms of expectations is **newfangled "miracle" surgery** or some sensational new machine you may hear about. There's the "weekend facelift" that supposedly does the work of a traditional facelift and healing takes a fraction of the time. Or the ad that says, "Have breast augmentation on the weekend and be back to work on Monday!" Needless to say, I am not just skeptical, but incredulous. I know these claims are physically impossible. You know what they say: if it sounds too good to be true...

So, what's new in liposuction? "Liposculpture" (sometimes also called selective, precision, fine, or micro liposuction) is small-volume sculpturing of areas previously not targeted for lipo—areas with less fat, like neck and facial areas, upper arms, along the spine, knees, and calves. These areas that are tricky for lipo because they have little fat, and it is fat needed for cushioning and contour, especially as we age. Some people do have problem areas that this technique can address, but it should be carefully considered.

I'm not saying one should not check out everything available, and there are new techniques being perfected every day. But I caution you to examine very carefully any new techniques. Remember, they have not been tried often, the kinks have yet to be worked out, and no one knows their long-term effects.

That is how the best surgeons handle new techniques. Of course, someone has to pioneer a procedure and do the research, but if the doctor you're talking to is not involved in doing that, find out just how long he has been doing a procedure. Prominent Los Angeles cosmetic surgeon Brian M. Kinney does just that. "When I see something come out and think it looks great, I wait probably somewhere between six months and a year to get into it. In my practice, one out of three or four of the things that come out, I will personally do. I can't do them all and I can trust my colleagues."

As you can see, a great way to steer clear of potentially risky techniques is to take the advice of an excellent surgeon. Good surgeons use good techniques. Stick with that, and you won't be sorry.

Have you heard about a Case Study?

If you think you can get cosmetic surgery for free by participating in a case study, you'd better think really hard about what you're getting into.

Case Study = Guinea Pig. Case studies are just what they say they are: you are a case and you are studied. Taking part in a case study means that you volunteer or are paid to be a guinea pig.

Personally, I am not an advocate of my clients being case studies when it comes to any kind of cosmetic procedures. A case study may entail a surgeon trying out a new technique or a new product on you, or it can be done for FDA approval of a product or device. Sometimes manufacturers or doctors will pay the patient over a period of time or do the operation for free.

In some fields of medicine, a case study may be appropriate for people who have no other choice, and the new procedure being tried could possibly improve or save their lives. I have a friend, for example, who had a very rare form of cancer. Her doctor knew of a case study being done using a new medication. She participated in the study, and her cancer is in remission. But it just as easily may not have worked. So, if you want to be a case study, just be forewarned—if the operation is not successful, even if it causes problems for the rest of you life, you have given permission for it and will not have much recourse.

Are you a good candidate?

Your surgeon will determine whether or not you are a good candidate physically for the procedure you want. He does this through testing, evaluation of your medical history, and discussion with you.

What we'll look at here are some ground rules I go by in helping people assess whether they are good candidates psychologically and attitude-wise.

- I've said it before and I'll say it again—cosmetic surgery will not change your life! If you're an angry person going in, you'll probably be an angry, slightly better contoured, person coming out.

- Having surgery won't mend a broken relationship, it won't win you a million dollars, and it won't get you a new job (unless maybe you're a lingerie model or a cross-dresser!).

- I don't recommend people have it to "keep up" with other people. Having your love handles lipoed because your boss had it done, or getting breast implants because they look great on your neighbor, doesn't make it right for you.

- If you have been through an emotionally distressing event, like divorce or the death of a loved one, give yourself a good amount of time (I recommend a year) to heal emotionally before having cosmetic surgery.

Truly good candidates are those who see the beginning signs of aging and want to halt them, or those who have something perceived as a flaw—like heavy eyelids, a protruding tummy, love handles—that they want to correct, and they know the procedure will fix that problem and nothing else.

Should you see a cosmetic surgery consultant?

Sometimes it can all be confusing and overwhelming. Perhaps you had no idea how complex it was to make a truly informed choice about liposuction—why and when to have it, what techniques to research, how to find the most qualified surgeon, how to prepare well, and how to recover most effectively. Whew! If you're taken aback by it all, a consultant may be right for you.

Why would someone even want to see a consultant before going forward with surgery? Well, think about why you use any kind of "broker" of services, such as a real estate agent or a car dealer or a financial planner. They are experts, the best of which can make things a whole lot simpler and more cost effective for you. Here's my favorite analogy: why use a travel expert? You know where you want to go, but you may not want to deal with the intricacies of getting the best value in tickets, hotels, and rental cars for the length of trip you're taking. Also, you'll probably be best served by an expert who has been there and can tell you the garden view at a particular resort is actually better than the ocean view, or that if you tip a certain amount on the first day you'll get better service throughout your stay.

Sometimes a cosmetic surgery consultant can help you with the initial decision of whether or not to pursue having liposuction. But more often, the consultant's role is to help you once you have decided you want something done. The consultant can provide lots of helpful information as well as referrals to qualified physicians, without you having to do all the homework and legwork. The more personalized a consultant's service is, the more you'll get out of it. For example, be wary if a service offers to provide you with referrals to doctors without first asking many questions about the results you are seeking.

As with other types of experts, a key to choosing the right cosmetic surgery consultant is finding someone with experience.

When I started having cosmetic work done, I had no one to advise me or answer my questions. I did the research into procedures on my own, investigated and interviewed physicians, and made certain to follow the recommendations about what to do before and after surgery. It took a lot of time and effort!

When I began my business, The Informed Choice, it was the first in the nation. Luckily, there are more of us today—people who learned about cosmetic surgery the hard way and are passing it along to make it easier and safer for others—like you!

The most important thing is to pick a cosmetic surgery consultant in a similar way to choosing a surgeon. Make sure the consultant you see is qualified and that the business is focused on helping you, the prospective patient. Criteria you should look for in a consultant include **track record** and **experience**. Here are some questions to ask:

How many people have they consulted? The number of times you hear about how someone recovers after liposuction or a brow lift does make a difference. After listening to individual experiences for more than 20 years, I know this has helped me to better prepare each new client.

So how does one get that experience? Well, I got mine through modeling and acting, where lots of folks I knew were having something done and sharing information about it. I was absolutely fascinated, and this led to further research and seeking out experts. Soon others were seeking me out for assistance, knowing that I'd had procedure after procedure with success and that I knew how to do my homework. Other consultants may have worked in a related field, for instance in a cosmetic surgeon's office, in beauty and fitness, or in a consultative healthcare role.

Be careful—some professed cosmetic surgery consultants claim broadly to have worked in "the healthcare field." Ask for specifics. This broad term can mean they were a dental hygienist, did bookkeeping for a chiropractor, or sold prostheses!

Have they had surgery themselves? And if so, have they had more than one procedure? Unfortunately, the world is full of people who have one facelift or get lipo of the thighs and—poof!—they are instant experts on the art and science of cosmetic surgery.

You should determine your level of comfort with the experience of the consultant, but remember that procedures and their associated challenges vary widely. Someone who has only had his or her eyes done won't be able to tell you how it feels to recover after a tummy tuck.

How do they choose the physicians to whom they refer? The answer you want to hear is that they do independent research, pick physicians with great track records and experience (the key is that they pick the doctors, the doctors don't come to them), and refer to physicians solely on the basis of qualifications and expertise—not because of a financial arrangement.

Also make sure you're paying the consultant for consulting service, while paying the surgeon for your procedure. A consultant should not be a middle person whom you pay for the operation.

To recap, make sure that the consultant is working on the consumer's behalf. What's important is that the consultant can give you detailed information about the doctors being recommended and clearly refers you to surgeons best at your particular procedure. If you simply receive a list of doctors and are told you can just go to any of them, then RUN, don't walk, to the nearest exit!

The Fear Factor:
How to Face Your Fears

Quite a few of my clients have told me that they've wanted to have cosmetic surgery for years. And for years, they have done nothing about it because they are afraid. Fear keeps many people from going forward with having a procedure done.

In this chapter, you'll learn what the most common fears tend to be, and I'll share some ways to help alleviate them if your ultimate goal is to have the procedure you want. The fears people have shared with me are discussed in the order of how common they are, with the most "popular" fear first.

Many times, a fear comes from what we don't know about something. Like nearly everything I tell you in this book, power comes from being informed. If you have the facts, you can often overcome fear in order to have a positive experience.

There are also fears people have after surgery. An important thing to remember is that paranoia (defined as unwarranted fear or delusion) can be an actual physical side effect of having surgery. If this happens, try to think back to what your fears, if any, were prior to surgery. If whatever you're afraid of now wasn't even an issue, it is likely a product of just such paranoia.

Anesthesia

By far the greatest fear most people have is that they will need to be under anesthesia during the operation. Usually, this stems from people not wanting to lose control. In some cases, people are simply afraid that once they are put under, they'll never wake up.

While anesthesia is usually the most dangerous aspect of having liposuction, complications of anesthesia have greatly declined in the past few decades. According to the American Society of Anesthesiologists, the number of anesthesiologists has more than doubled since 1970, and patient outcomes have improved at about the same rate. Over the last 10 years, the number of deaths attributable to anesthesia (during any type of operation) has dropped from 1 in 10,000 to 1 in 250,000.

I've offered my clients some advice that seems to help:

- Think about how many people you know who actually have not woken up from surgery. You probably don't know of any. It is extremely rare today for anesthesia to be the cause of death.

- Remember, there are people in hospitals around the country and the world every day undergoing surgery under twilight and general anesthesia. And some of these people are having operations for serious conditions, such as open-heart surgery, and they do just fine.

- If the thought of going under anesthesia scares you, you need to talk to the anesthesiologist or nurse anesthetist about your fear. He or she can tell you how things will work and assure you about being there with you throughout the entire operation. (If possible, try to talk to the anesthesiologist well ahead of the operation; in some cases, one may not be assigned until the day before.)

- You may also be afraid of getting sick after waking from the anesthesia, which can be a side effect. Again, talk to the anesthesiologist. There are ways (including a pill or a shot) to help lower the chances of this happening. If you have had bouts of vomiting following anesthesia in the past, or you have a fear of this happening, express this strongly to your surgeon.

Some people fear waking up in the middle of the operation. This can conceivably happen, but it is very rare. If you have this fear, discuss it well ahead of time with the anesthesiologist. Keep in mind that drinking and drug use can impact the ability of the anesthesia medication to put you under and keep you under. If you have used drugs or alcohol in the 24-hour period before your operation, or may have drugs in your system from extensive use, you need to be upfront with your surgeon and anesthesiologist about this. Remember that it's all confidential (by law!), and it is for your own well-being and safety.

Bad results

Some people don't venture into cosmetic surgery because they are afraid that their results won't be what they want. They may hear horror stories about botched operations, or they may simply invent the worst-case scenario in their own minds.

If you feel you have...

- interviewed enough surgeons

- chosen the most qualified doctor

- communicated to him in every way (verbally and visually) what results you want, and what you *don't* want

...then, stop worrying!

An important factor is that you be realistic about what a bad result is. One example of a truly poor result is ending up with one side of the liposuctioned area noticeably smaller, larger, or otherwise uneven from the other—like having one hip look larger than the other! That really is unacceptable, of course, and the surgeon would need to fix it. Remember, this unlikely to happen if the doctor is experienced and qualified.

Don't be too quick to judge your results as poor, either. It's very important to keep in mind how long recovery takes and that the ultimate result of your liposuction may take months to emerge. Every procedure goes through a series of changes during healing. Be sure to listen to your surgeon about what is normal during this process.

> A couple of weeks after I had upper and lower blepharoplasty (eye job), the bruising had dissipated and I was healing well. Then one morning, I woke up and almost fell over when I looked in the mirror.

> One eye was big and round like a marble, and the other was almond-shaped and squinty. I freaked! Hysterical and in tears, I called my girlfriend Randi, who had had an eye job herself and was a good and honest friend.

> "Girl," she screamed, "get away from that mirror!" She assured me that it was just the swelling and that days like this might pop up for a while. I checked this with the doctor's office (as you should do if concerned about something), and they agreed. My best bet was to not to keep tracking progress in the mirror, especially in the morning when most people are a little puffy.

Sure enough, it flip-flopped the next day, with the previously round eye appearing squinty. This went on for about a month, with some days being better than others. Most importantly, this experience became a turning point for me. I realized there are things people really need to know that are not described, at least not well enough, in the doctor's office. It isn't that the surgeon and his staff aren't doing a good job; it's just that there is *so much* to know! It's scary enough having changes like this happen when you *know* ahead of time that they might. But being prepared can certainly ease the fear. (That's why you're reading this book, so you'll be as prepared as you can be.)

If there is a problem, get a clear answer from your surgeon ahead of time about whether it can be treated, how it would be fixed, and when. It helps to ease the fear when you know something can be fixed. For example, if there is not quite enough fat removed during liposuction, you can always have more removed during a second procedure. On the other hand, what can't be fixed is too much fat being taken out, causing dimpling and saggy skin. The moral of this story? Less is better, as a rule of thumb. You can always have additional procedures, but it's hard to go backwards, and sometimes impossible to put something back once it's gone. For some severe cases, doctors have found ways to transfer fat, but it's far more trouble and expense than having lipo a little at a time to achieve the look you desire.

Complications and risks

Similar to fears about bad results are fears of something unpredictable going wrong.

It is normal to be fearful when you're told about the risks of surgery, no matter how remote they may be. You'll be told about a great many possible risks, some of which are extremely rare—in fact, some may never happen, but in theory they could. You're given all this information so that you can make a choice for yourself about whether to go forward.

Certain risk factors can be another story. If you are at risk for a particular complication because of your body type or skin type, lifestyle, habits, a medical condition, or prior injuries or operations, you have reason to be cautious. You need to discuss all of the risks with your doctor. If he tells you are at high risk for a particular complication, take it seriously. (If one doctor tells you it's not that big a risk, while others are saying to be careful, it may be a sign that the *doctor* is willing to take the risk…but it's your health he's risking!)

If you are simply paralyzed by fear, the answer is simple: don't have surgery. You need to be comfortable and have a positive outlook to obtain the results you want and deserve. Your fear will cause stress, which takes a physical toll. The healing process can be hard enough without your mind working against it.

People finding out

Some people's biggest fear is that they will have all the "white lies" down, they'll take enough time off, and they'll camouflage the swelling and bruising—and someone might still come up to them and say, "So, you had some liposuction done!"

You have to allow for the possibility that someone could peg what you had done. Usually, these are very visual people or those who have had the same procedure. Then you'll need to decide if they are trustworthy and you can confide in them and ask for their cooperation in keeping your secret, or if you'll need to wiggle out of it with more white lies. One way I have found that works well for many people is to not quite say whether you've had something done:

> *Your friend:* "Have you had something done to your hips? Did you actually have liposuction?"
>
> *You:* "Why do you ask?"
>
> *Your friend:* "Well, you look different..."
>
> *You:* "A lot of people have said that. I've been taking good care of myself, working out a lot, and eating right. I thought it was time, and I guess it's working!"

The truth was told ... just not the whole truth!

Also, remember when I mentioned paranoia at the beginning of this chapter? Part of what a procedure can bring about is that people swear others are staring at them all the time. This perception may be just an aftereffect of surgery.

Or it may be that they *are* staring, but they're doing so because you look *great*! The more pudgy you are before liposuction, the greater the difference will be, and people are bound to take a second look. They probably won't know that you had lipo, however; they will think you've lost weight and spent lots of time in the gym.

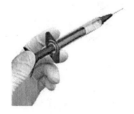

Needles

Don't be embarrassed about being afraid of needles. It's very common. Be upfront about it, and try to tell the doctor and his staff specifically what you're afraid of. Did you have a bad experience with someone not being able to find a vein? Does the thought of having a shot make you faint?

If you are about to have surgery, needles are unavoidable. You'll have to have a shot to numb the area where your IV will be put in. Talk about what scares you so that the surgical team can be especially sensitive about these issues. Remember, your doctor wants a satisfied patient, so you'll get what you need to the best of his ability.

Fear itself

Fright. Bad attitude. Negative thoughts. I include these as a separate discussion because they are so important.

The mind is an unbelievably powerful thing. Think about studies in which patients given placebos experience similar effects as those given actual medications—that's the power of the mind!

Going into the whole cosmetic surgery experience with a bad attitude, unreasonable fears, or negative thoughts can actually *cause* complications. It's one thing to be informed and truly consider possible risks and complications, but it's another thing altogether to work yourself into a tizzy over possibilities that may never become a problem.

The best way to allay fears and bad thoughts is to be informed about your procedure. This means reading and talking to those qualified to provide good information. I seriously doubt you'll find the best information in a chat room! Once you've done your homework, stop worrying, and KNOW that you'll have the best experience if you visualize the best results possible. **What you focus on will be more likely to happen.**

It is also really important to surround yourself with positive people before, during, and after surgery. Avoid those with negative things to say about what you're having done. They can erode your good feelings about your procedure, and you'll need those during the healing process.

Doctors

Some people have a problem even getting to the point of finding a good surgeon because they are so intimidated by doctors. If this is you, please read the next chapter about doctors. This is one fear it is absolutely critical you put aside if you're going to find the best person to perform your surgery. Read the next chapter NOW!

Doctors...Physicians ...Surgeons... Oh, my! Let's take the "doc" off his pedestal.

I have a friend who—well, there's no other way to put it—can barely take care of himself. Over the past several years, I have tried to help him learn to cook simple meals, wash his clothes, and do small repairs around his home. It's no use. He will probably always eat out, visit the Chinese laundry, and pay a handyman to change his light bulbs. When I tell him something is easy to do, he replies, "Yeah, maybe for you!"

Funny thing is, this same man is a highly skilled and very talented surgeon who has successfully operated on thousands of patients. For him, performing surgery is not that difficult; he is trained and has done the operations he performs over and over.

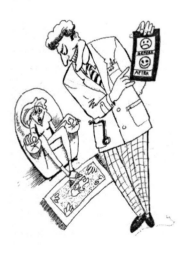

Why do I tell you this story? I want to point out that we all have various talents, were raised differently, learned distinct skills, and became good at diverse things. We look to others to help us do the things we can't, and the things that we elected not to study in school. A lawyer takes care of our legal matters, a mechanic fixes our car, and a stay-at-home mom can care for the kids and get everything done around the house in ways that might overwhelm her career-oriented friend! For many of us, doing what these people do would be very difficult, if not impossible.

Doctors are people, too

Why do doctors intimidate us? Simply, because we let them. Our society has positioned doctors as "god-like" because they can save lives, make us stop hurting, or help us look prettier or thinner. Who wouldn't think that's the greatest ability on earth? They are intelligent people who have gone through an intensive educational process and are skilled in what they practice. But just like the architect we hire to design a house, or the accountant we pay to do our taxes, the surgeon is performing the job for which we employ him.

Webster's Dictionary defines intimidation as "to make timid or fearful." These are responses that don't serve us well when we are trying to make an important choice. The good news is, they can be avoided.

Certainly, doctors who do exceptional work in their particular field deserve a great deal of respect. By all means, show respect, but don't let yourself become paralyzed by fear or awe when you speak with surgeons. For people who feel this level of anxiety, I suggest they look at the surgeon as a person they hire to do a job. Good ways to avoid the consequences of nervousness include

- **being informed** about what you want to have done
- **writing down questions** that you want to ask a doctor
- trying some **relaxation techniques** before a doctor's appointment: breathe deeply, do a meditation exercise, or think of your favorite place—whatever helps you feel more comfortable.

Two doctors are better than one

An important concept about choosing your surgeon is that you actually have choices. **Getting only one opinion is a big-time NO-NO!**

Think about it: if you decided to renovate your house, wouldn't you interview more than one contractor before you lay down your money for the work? Don't you want the best person for the assignment, one with whom you can communicate and who understands what results that you want?

Well, what you're doing through liposuction is renovating your face or body. You'll be living with the results for a long time, so you want the most qualified person for the job.

Let's face it; trying to find the right doctor is confusing.

It's hard to know who to trust and whose advice to take, to be satisfied that you have enough information, and to feel you're making the right decision. If it all gets to be too much, I do recommend that you seek advice from a cosmetic surgery consultant who can recommend surgeons. Just as you might consult *Consumers Digest* before you purchase a major appliance, remember that those of us who have made it our career to help you with these choices are here for you. We know the industry and have done the homework and legwork, so you don't have to. Just as you'd do when choosing a doctor, be sure to check out the reputability of the consultants you consider. Read more about using a cosmetic surgery consultant on pages 36–39.

Carol's Top Five Physician Fiascos

Here is a list of mistakes that people make when it comes to doctors. It has grown pretty naturally out of the experiences I've had over the years. What can I say, except that they should be avoided like the plague! Making sure that these potential problems don't trip you up can help you have the positive cosmetic surgery experience you deserve.

#1 "I don't have the time to get more than one opinion."

WRONG ANSWER! You *need* to get more than one opinion, and I recommend three.

> A physician's assistant, about 45, once came to see me after having poorly done eyelid surgery. She had gone to one doctor, had the surgery, was very unhappy, and was getting nowhere with having her complaints addressed. The doctor was probably not qualified in the first place, which she would have known if she had done her research and talked with several physicians. This patient—in the medical professional herself— should have known better, you may say. Well, the point is that anyone can make a mistake.

Avoid common pitfalls, and hiring the first doctor you meet is one of them. *Always* interview more than one surgeon.

#2 "My friend said this doctor is great."

That's wonderful. By all means, add his name to your list of doctors to interview. But don't let that be your only compass. Why does your friend recommend him? Were they old college buddies, or did this surgeon actually perform your friend's procedure? Even if he did—and your friend looks great—remember that you are unique. You may not be as good a candidate for surgery, may not heal as fast, or may not even need the same type of procedure. Do your own research and decide on the merits of what YOU need and want.

#3 "I'm embarrassed to talk to the doctor about that."

Then you might as well forget it until you get your courage up. That may sound harsh, but I want to make the point that you need to talk to your doctor about lots of things—before and after your procedure—and you *must* curb your fear, embarrassment, and intimidation if you're going to get the results you want. Before liposuction, you will need to share medical history and even some personal information so the procedure can be done effectively and safely. And afterwards, you have to tell your doctor if you're experiencing anything questionable during recovery. At any point, don't be afraid to question the doctor. He wants you to be a satisfied patient, and if you're not happy, you need to tell him. How else will he know...unless he's psychic?

#4 "I can't wait to have this surgery—I'll finally be happy!"

If you plan to have cosmetic surgery to "fix your life," don't do it. It won't mend a relationship, it won't give you better friends, and it won't land you a great new job. And if you go into it with expectations like these, you are setting yourself up for major disappointment.

> I had a wealthy female client once who wanted to have a series of procedures to counter the effects of aging and enable her to compete with her husband's young girlfriend. I stopped the consultation. She was not considering having surgery for herself; looks were not even her problem. It was a case for a marriage

counselor, not a cosmetic surgeon. Luckily, she decided against going through the time, expense, and pain of surgery—all of which *she*, not her husband, would have endured.

#5 "My doctor says I should rest another week, but I really want to go on this trip."

Not taking your doctor's advice is unacceptable. Cosmetic surgery is just that—surgery—and ignoring warnings about what you should and shouldn't do before or after surgery has its consequences. I'll explain some of the things you may need to be careful about in the sections about preparing for and recovering from liposuction. While these are great things for you to know, keep in mind that you are unique, and your doctor's advice will be geared toward you, your lifestyle and health, the way you heal, and your specific procedure.

Who is qualified to perform your surgery?

The last 10 years or so have seen a "Cosmetic Surgery Gold Rush." Cosmetic techniques have become incredibly popular, with nearly 11.5 million surgical and non-surgical procedures performed in 2006 in the United States alone. Since 1997, when collection of the statistics first began, surgical procedures have increased 123% and nonsurgical procedures 749%.[1] A combination of factors has brought out the best, and the worst. An aging population who want to stay looking as young as they feel has intersected with the rise of managed care, making cosmetic surgery a lucrative field for physicians. This brings out the best because procedures are done more often, perfecting surgical techniques and decreasing risks. It brings out the

---

1 Statistics are courtesy of the American Society for Aesthetic Plastic Surgery.

worse because there are always those who want to cash in on a Gold Rush—and you don't want to be the first Monday morning liposuction appointment of an internist who just took a weekend course…

Just as you would not ask a mechanic who specializes in repairing German cars to fix something on a Honda, you want to be sure the doctor you choose to perform your surgery truly specializes in liposuction. While the German car mechanic probably could repair the Honda, and maybe even do a great job, wouldn't you feel better knowing the person working on your Honda had the experience of working on many others, knew all the intricacies of its particular engine, and had the right parts to make it run well again? The same is true for cosmetic surgery: Just because a doctor can perform a variety of procedures, it does not mean he has the amount of experience you want for your liposuction.

If you're like most people, you probably have found a family physician you see regularly. Because you trust your doctor, he may be one of the first people you ask for advice as you begin to think about having cosmetic surgery. It's a good place to start, but I'm going to give you some guidelines about what kind of advice to take from whom, and how to weight it all in making the right choice for *you*.

The first thing I caution you about is that any doctor with a medical license can take a course in cosmetic surgery and hang a shingle that says he performs cosmetic procedures. This is why knowing a doctor's actual background—including credentials and experience—is so important in separating out those qualified to best meet your needs. The bottom line is, the doctor you choose for your cosmetic procedure should be trained and experienced in just that: cosmetic surgery. If you do approach a physician in a specialty other than cosmetic surgery to perform your procedure, at least be sure that he has performed the surgery before and that his specialty is related to what you want to have done, such as a plastic/ reconstructive surgeon, who normally operates to fix deformities caused by birth defects or accidents, being qualified to perform aesthetic cosmetic surgery.

Also check the section at the back of this book for a list of medical boards. There, you can read more about which board certifications qualify surgeons to perform which procedures.

Who is "the best?"

You've probably heard of quite a few cosmetic surgeons. Even if you don't know their names, you certainly have read or heard about some of their famous patients. Think about the nips and tucks that have graced the headlines, like those of Pamela Anderson, Sharon Osbourne, Demi Moore, Michael Douglas, and Britney Spears. The list is way too long to include here!

How do some surgeons become famous? Are the famous ones the best? Not necessarily. Some surgeons are known for their famous patients. High-priced doctors can hire high-priced PR people to spread the word about them. There are locally famous surgeons everywhere. They may be known for making the mayor's wife look 20 years younger, or they may be great philanthropists, or they may be respected for reconstructive work they do for the people who could not otherwise afford surgery. They might even be known for their spectacular golf game!

The point is, like any other profession, individuals may get a reputation—good or bad—based on people talking about them, for whatever reason. The moral of the story? The famous doctor in question may indeed be the best. But don't go by fame alone—just because a doctor has operated on a celebrity or done something else that has started tongues wagging does not necessarily mean he is the best surgeon to perform your procedure.

Red Flag #1: If a doctor or his office staff spreads the news about who has been in his office, you need to wonder about the level of confidentiality you'll receive.

You can barely open a magazine these days without seeing the slick ads of cosmetic surgeons, all saying "I'm the best!" They certainly have a lot of confidence. That's good—you want a surgeon who is sure of himself. But they can't ALL be "the best." How do you find the truth? *Do your homework, ask questions, and keep your eyes and ears open!*

Some people ask whether they should travel out of their area or out of the country to have cosmetic surgery. If you live in a rural or remote area where there are no practicing or qualified cosmetic surgeons, the answer is, of course, yes—go where you find the best surgeon for your needs. But chances are, especially with the boom in this field, that there are good surgeons located near you. Many people are under the impression that to have the best surgeon and get the best care, they need to travel to a perceived cosmetic surgery "Mecca" like Los Angeles, New York, or even South America.

Rubbish!

It's true that in some places—like the movie capital of Los Angeles or the modeling hub of New York—there is high demand for cosmetic surgery and, therefore, doctors in these areas see more patients. That does not mean, however, that they are any more skilled or talented than surgeons practicing in your city. It's also important to remember the added costs, in both money and time, that traveling will mean.

Similarly, some people believe that great results can be guaranteed by paying a high price. They may gravitate to the "elite," higher-priced doctors.

Baloney!

Sometimes, all that those higher prices mean is that the doctor has higher overhead, like a nice big office, on-site surgical suites, and lots of equipment. Or maybe he just bought a penthouse and a Mercedes convertible! I have come across doctors in various parts of the country who finance everything from race cars to yachts to private planes through their practice. This is not to say there's anything inherently wrong with that—if someone is successful, he should reap the rewards of his labors—but as a patient advocate, it's my role to tell you that higher price does not necessarily mean better results. And vice-versa, cut rates also don't mean better value.

Finding good doctors

Choosing the best surgeon to perform your procedure is probably the single most important factor to getting the results you want. Your choice should come after careful decision-making and weighing factors such as the doctor's credentials and experience, convenience and pricing, and how comfortable you are with the surgeon (after all, you will be seeing quite a bit of each other from pre-op to surgery and throughout the recovery process). Your decision will be based on finding out these factors and comparing several physicians. This is why the interview process is so important. I emphatically recommend that, if you do nothing else, you should interview at least three surgeons, but not more than five. I'll explain the reasons for this later in this chapter.

Most importantly, you need to know the questions to ask and the answers to seek. You have to know that the surgeon you choose is qualified, has the experience and credentials to perform your procedure, knows the risk potential for this operation, and takes appropriate steps to make it as safe as possible.

On the whole, most surgeons are good and aim for the best results for their patients. The key is to ferret out the occasional ones that are not so good and those who are downright quacks. But once you know you are dealing with good ones, you also need to heed their advice.

To emphasize this, I have to tell you a story at this point that, very unfortunately, is true. And it is perhaps the most important reason that I do what I do to help people make safe and informed choices, so that nothing like this happens to anyone else.

> In 1998, I got a call in my office. I remember that day. It was a woman with a warm, genuine voice. Her name was Judy Loveless. "I've seen lots of things written about you," she said, "how you help people who are thinking about cosmetic surgery. I liked what I read. I'd really like to get together and talk."

> We set a date and kept chatting. She was a flight attendant, had been for 20 years. She'd flown millions of miles. And we all know what a toll that can take.

> "Just being on the ground for 20 years can take a toll," I said. We both laughed.

> She was in her late 40s, she said, but later when I saw a photo, she easily looked 10 years younger. She was

gorgeous, with short brown hair and a lovely smile. The day we talked, she said she'd had several procedures—breasts, eyes, a facelift—and just wanted to talk to someone neutral that she could trust about cosmetic surgery. She never mentioning she was thinking about having one more procedure. She later called to reschedule for a future date.

Six weeks later, the phone rang again.

"Don't you know Judy Loveless?" It was Dr. Vincent Zubowicz of Atlanta, whom she'd recently asked to do laser resurfacing on her face to take away some fine wrinkles and smooth out the skin. He'd explained to her how it worked: with a pencil-sized tool, a sort of magic wand that emits a laser beam, the doctor burns off a layer of skin and brand new skin grows back— with fewer lines. "But I recommended she didn't need it," he said. "She went to someone else."

"So did she get it done?" I asked.

"You don't know?" he asked.

"Know what?"

"She's dead."

For a minute, I could hardly breathe, still remembering our talk. She had been like someone you meet for the first time but feel you've known all your life.

"What happened?" I couldn't believe the story I heard. And I heard it many more times as it erupted in headlines and on TV.

Two qualified surgeons advised her she didn't need the procedure, but she had done it anyway. She ended up going to a clinic in a strip mall. The doctor there, an ophthalmologist who had recently added cosmetic procedures to his repertoire, had said "no problem" and did it in the office. Under anesthesia, her blood pressure dropped. There were no monitors to show this; there were no medications on hand to reverse it; there was no emergency equipment to revive her. The doctor called an ambulance. They sped Judy to the hospital, but she died.

Later, the board of medical examiners determined the doctor and clinic had failed to provide a safe place for surgery. Even though many routine operations are done safely every day in physicians' offices, this clinic failed to provide for an emergency. The doctor surrendered his license and was charged with manslaughter. The clinic was sued for malpractice. But none of that will bring Judy back.

I was heartbroken about a woman I'd never met—and I was angry. It's haunted me ever since. If she'd only told me what she was thinking about, I could have given her questions to ask to make sure the doctor was board-certified and qualified, that his office was safe and prepared to handle anything that might happen during surgery, that he'd done this many times with great success, and more.

Well, I can't help Judy anymore, but I can tell everyone else considering cosmetic surgery what they need to ask and listen for when seeking the surgeon into whose hands they will place themselves.

The rest of this chapter explains how to find the best surgeon for you, step by step. The focus is on how to assess specific criteria about the doctor himself, credentials and experience, the surgical facility, pricing, and even office staff.

Choosing the best surgeon for you

Step 1: Find several good doctors

Become a sleuth, or think like an investigative reporter. Finding potential doctors to interview can be done in several ways:

Directories

A good place to begin can be the Marquis *Official ABMS Directory of Board Certified Medical Specialists*. Check your local library. Keep in mind are that volumes like this can help you start a list of doctors to check out, but they become quickly outdated and don't provide any value judgment about who does what best.

Ask your primary physician

Doctors talk to one another, and most know what's going on in their profession locally. Asking your family doctor or other physicians you know for information about who they think is best for specific procedures can be fruitful. One suggestion is that you dig deeper when provided with a name—do they know the skills and experience of the surgeon they recommend, or are they only acquainted socially? If a doctor tells you he knows a particular cosmetic surgeon is really good, don't be afraid to ask how he knows! It is also important to know if the recommended doctor is experienced in the specific procedure you're considering. He may be great at doing breasts but not liposuction.

Check with local hospitals

You can call local hospitals where plastic or reconstructive surgery is performed and ask for the name of the surgeon who serves as their Chief of Plastic Surgery. It's a good bet that a doctor named to such a position at a reputable hospital is well qualified. Then call his office and find out what percentage of his surgery is cosmetic surgery or liposuction specifically. If it is none to very little, keep looking. My advice is that you should find a surgeon who does at least 50% cosmetic surgery. This will mean that this doctor is a good candidate for your list of surgeons to interview.

Query friends who have had cosmetic surgery

It's OK to get the name of the cosmetic surgeon who did such a great facelift for your cousin Chris. As in any business, satisfied customers are a great measure of good work. A very big caution here, however, is that a personal recommendation must not keep you from doing due diligence to the process of making your choice. Interview this surgeon as you would any other. Is the procedure he did so well for someone else the same as what you want done? And remember that one person's successful outcome doesn't guarantee yours will be the same.

Board certified surgeons list

You can contact the American Board of Plastic Surgery for a list of surgeons in your area. Depending on the procedure you're having, there are other boards you will want to contact. Check out the Medical Boards section at the back of this book. You can also access listings of surgeons and their credentials on the Internet.

Referral services

If there is a personalized cosmetic surgery information and referral service in your area, it may be your safest, fastest, easiest, and most effective means of ensuring you have a successful and satisfying experience. I've told you a little about my company, The Informed Choice. Its whole reason for being is to help people who are considering cosmetic surgery in making a decision, choosing a qualified doctor, preparing and recovering well, and getting answers to all the questions that inevitably come up. And I have the experience to provide the peace of mind my clients seek during this process. If there is a similar service this in your area, I suggest you look into it and—finding it reputable and focused on your needs—utilize it to make things easier on yourself! Face-to-face is the best way to have a cosmetic surgery consultant assist you, but if that's not possible, keep in mind that The Informed Choice offers telephone consultations. (See pages 36–39 for ways to find a qualified consultant.)

Step 2: Narrow down the list

Next, narrow down your choice of surgeons based on what you may know or find out about the doctors on your list. For example, you may hear positive feedback from someone who had surgery performed by a specific surgeon, and—although you will be careful to choose based on your OWN needs—this may place him on the "Definitely Interview" list. Or, you may discover that another surgeon operates very far from where you live, and this may move him further down on your list. (But don't get too hung up on location; remember the most important aspect to choosing your physician is his qualifications.)

Now you should have your "A List" of three physicians who will be the first doctors you will interview. It doesn't mean you can't keep going after that. It's an important decision about your body—make sure you are 100% sure that you're making a choice with which you're comfortable.

Interview three surgeons but not more than five. Why? Common sense and the "Law of Averages." Let me explain:

On the minimum end, I am adamant that my clients take the time and make the effort to see three doctors before choosing one to perform their procedure. To make an informed decision, you need to have information and you need to have choices, and talking to only one possible surgeon is not a choice. The interview process is vital because you'll find out in person things that no one else can tell you, like how well a doctor listens to *you* and understands what *you* really expect from your procedure.

On the maximum end, I've seen people go overboard with how many surgeons they interview before making a decision. One former client kept interviewing doctors until she had seen *eleven*! She spent a lot of time and money on a decision she apparently wasn't ready to make. I strongly recommend that if you have not found a surgeon with whose qualifications and demeanor you are satisfied after meeting with five doctors, you need to reexamine the issues: is surgery really what you want, is this the right time, and do you have realistic expectations of the results? The need to keep seeing more doctors—because none are telling you what you want to hear about how the procedure might turn out, or because they are recommending you not have surgery—is a warning sign that you need to reconsider.

Step 3: Meet at least three surgeons

Once you have your "A List," make appointments to see these doctors to discuss your desired procedure. Remember, you're thinking about hiring one of these surgeons and paying him a lot of money. Make sure to discover why you should

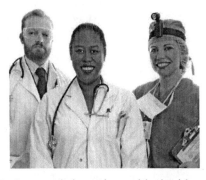

pick one over the others. Go into each interview with the idea of having the doctor "sell himself" to you—not the other way around. The question on your mind should be, "What can you do for me?"

When you call to schedule appointments, be aware that most surgeons, though not all, charge a pre-surgical consultation fee, ranging from $50 to $400 (in big cities, the fees will be closer to the high end). Basically, you're paying for their valuable time, materials you will receive about the procedure, and computerized imaging they may use to give you an idea of the "before and after" possibilities of your procedure.

One of the advantages of making your "A List" after visiting a cosmetic surgery consultant is that many surgeons waive their interview appointment fee for prospective patients referred by a cosmetic surgery consultant. Since you can usually receive up to three referrals from the consultant, this can save you two thirds or more of what you would have paid for these consultations. The reason physicians often waive the fee for referrals from cosmetic surgery consultants is because they know they are getting informed individuals in their office, ones who will ask the right questions and not waste their time.

Step 4: The interview

The most important aspect of the interview is being prepared. **Have your questions written down!** Do not jot them down in the reception area before you see the doctor or in your car on the way to his office. Start writing down questions as soon as you make the decision to set an appointment.

As you prepare for each doctor interview, keep a notebook with you and write down further questions as they come to you. I have found that most doctors welcome questions and have stated that consultations are more productive for both parties when the patient brings in prepared questions.

To help you get started, I've included an interview checklist at the end of this chapter (pages 92 to 94); be sure to add your own questions.

Typically, this pre-surgical consultation will begin with the office staff providing you with some general information and materials and probably having you fill out information for their files. The information you receive should include the surgeon's CV, short for *curriculum vitae*, the equivalent of a resume for doctors. This may answer many of the general questions about the doctor's background, such as where he attended medical school and completed residency, what board certifications he holds, and where he has hospital privileges. While you're waiting to see the surgeon, look through the materials and check off any questions on your list answered in them so that you won't ask the doctor about them again. You can spend your time more wisely delving deeper into whether he's the right surgeon for you.

> **Red Flag #2:** If the surgeon doesn't seem to like you asking questions or avoids answering them to your satisfaction, perhaps you need to look for a different surgeon.

Be aware that consultations for different procedures can take different amounts of time. For example, a small-area liposuction interview will be relatively short (maybe 15 or 20 minutes), whereas an appointment to discuss multiple facial procedures or large-volume liposuction can take quite a bit longer, as there is much more to talk about.

Here are some important questions that you should ask each physician you interview. These should help you start your list. Just as important as asking these questions is truly listening to the answers you get and watching the reaction to each question.

Questions to Ask about Your Procedure

- *How long is the recovery for this procedure?*

    Some of the standard recovery times are provided for you in the liposuction chapter. It is a good idea to discuss your surgeon's recommendations. Keep in mind that it is always a better idea to plan more time than not enough.

- *What are the risks involved with my procedure?*

    There are risks to every operation. That's a fact. Look for honesty. The surgeon should tell you what might happen, no matter how slim the chance. Now, more than likely there will be no risk of eye injury when you're having liposuction of the tummy, but you get the point!

- *What types of complications are associated with this procedure?*

  If a doctor says, "I never have complications," look at his nose—you just might see it grow a foot or two. While it's true that some people heal well and don't encounter any complications, there are some problems inherent to liposuction. The surgeon should explain when a problem is considered a complication and how it is addressed.

- *If I have a complication, can it be corrected, and at what point will it be corrected?*

  Many complications are not recognized as such until a reasonable amount of healing time has passed. For example, you'll want to know when scar revision might be performed if an incision point does not heal well—in three months, six months, longer?

- *If I would need to undergo surgery a second time, is there a second fee? Will there be an additional charge for the operating room and anesthesia?*

  There usually is not a fee for the doctor to perform a corrective procedure, but there are charges for the operating room, anesthesia, medications, and so on. Be aware that, if you lose your mind and start eating like a hog, thereby gaining weight, the doctor may not do touch-up lipo until you are back to your original weight (where you were when you first had lipo).

- *Will my healing time be longer because the area has been operated on twice?*

  This varies by procedure. Have the doctor explain.

- *Are there alternatives to the procedures I want to have done?*

Sometimes there are other ways to achieve your desired outcome, besides what you had in mind. For example, you might go in thinking you need a little liposuction for a potbelly but what you really need is a tummy tuck.

- *Will you* (the doctor to whom you're speaking) *be the one performing the surgery?*

Sometimes doctors have fellows or residents in training working under them (remember, they all had to start somewhere!). Though residents are dedicated to their craft and closely supervised by the attending physician, it is up to you whether you want one of these physicians to work on you.

- *Is it possible to talk to some former patients about the experiences they had with this procedure?*

A doctor may have some patients who have given permission to talk to others, but remember that in this day and age of HIPAA[2] regulations, privacy is paramount. Even if the doctor does know of a willing patient, you probably won't get a name that day, as he'll have to check with the patient first. Also keep in mind that you won't be getting the name of anyone who was not happy with the procedure.

- *Will you be available to me after my liposuction?*

It is not unusual for doctors to perform several operations one week, then take a few weeks off and possibly take a vacation. Many people are OK with this (after all, doctors have to have lives, too), but it's best if you know he won't

---

2 **HIPAA:** the Health Insurance Portability and Accountability Act of 1996, a group of privacy, security, and coding regulations for the healthcare industry

be there and find out ahead of time whom you'll be dealing with for any questions or problems you encounter.

- *Where will the incision(s) be made?*

Although this varies with what type of lipo you're having done—and any accompanying procedure—it is always important to be aware of exactly where your incisions will be. The doctor will probably discuss this with you, but sometimes if you don't ask, the doctor may assume that you already know. I can't tell how many times people have told me, "I didn't know the incision would be **there**!"

- *Can you do my liposuction in a hospital, and if so, which one?*

Some liposuction can be done in a doctor's office or surgical suite, and other procedures are routinely done in a hospital setting. Regardless of this, the surgeon should be able to admit patients to a good hospital, should the need arise. Rule of thumb: good hospitals have good doctors. Find out where the doctor has privileges and whether those include surgery. You can call the hospital to confirm.

Questions to Ask the Surgeon about His Training

- *What board certification(s) do you have?*

See the back of the book for more information about medical boards and certifications.

When you are conducting interviews, it is very positive if a doctor is a member of ASPS (American Society of Plastic Surgeons) and/or a member of (ASAPS) American Society for Aesthetic Plastic Surgery, as these organizations have stringent requirements for member doctors (including board certification). If the surgeon is not part of these, ask why. Then listen for good answers!

- *How long have you been board-certified?*

  When a surgeon finishes residency, he is then officially a doctor, ready to practice. He must practice under the same roof for two years before he can take board exams, which involves submitting all of the operations he has done and taking written and oral examinations. If a surgeon does a fellowship after his residency, he can't realistically be studying for board exams at the same time. Others get so busy in their practice, they find it hard to take time for the exam. All this is to say that you want to find a board-certified physician, even if certification is recent.

- *How long have you been performing cosmetic surgery?*

  My opinion is that a doctor who has done a cosmetic surgery fellowship (which means six months to a year of concentration in nothing but cosmetic surgery) is more advanced earlier on. Others may have had no fellowship but may have done liposuction for 10 years. Still others may not have as much experience but have a natural talent. The bottom line is that you have to be personally comfortable with what you find out.

- *What percentage of your work is cosmetic surgery?*

  Again, your comfort level is important here. I recommend 50% of a surgeon's work be cosmetic. If you find a great doctor who usually does something other than cosmetic surgery but performs lipo a few dozen times a year, you may elect to have him do it. Many doctors, however, do nothing but cosmetic surgery and understand the unique issues associated with it.

- *What kind of experience have you had with the procedure I want? How many times have you performed this operation? Are there different ways to do it? Which do you prefer, and why?*

Remember that some procedures are more popular than others (see the chart on page 81). If you're having a popular procedure, and a doctor you speak with has not done many, you can be sure there are other surgeons out there who have. Conversely, be realistic about how many of a less-often-done procedure he could possibly have preformed.

Questions to Ask about the Doctor's Office

- *What is your policy about confidentiality? What about the staff?*

The answer you want is that your rights to privacy are absolute! You'll be asked whether your before-and-after photos can be used for potential patients to see, and possibly about talking with future patients about your results. Remember it's OK to say no. Regarding office staff, watch and listen: Do they drop names casually? Are they careful about patient names being seen or heard by others in the office?

- *If I decide I would like you to perform the procedure, where would it be done?*

Some procedures are safely done in the doctor's office with certain precautions, while others require a fully staffed operating room (OR). In either case, make sure the operating room is accredited by AAAHC (Accreditation Association for Ambulatory Health Care, Inc.), or AAAASF (American Association for Accreditation of Ambulatory Surgical Facilities), or JCAHO (Joint Commission on Accreditation of Healthcare Organization). Hospital ORs always are accredited, but a doctor's office OR may not be. Request to see the accreditation certificate, evidence that the facility meets high standards of safety and patient care. This accreditation also verifies that the surgeon is licensed and board-certified, all other personnel (nursing staff, anesthetists, etc.) are highly trained and certified, and the facility has state-of-the-art instruments and monitoring equipment. You can also request to see the OR. Does it have what's needed for patient safety (crash cart, defibrillator, monitoring equipment, drugs)? Is the Patient Bill of Rights posted?

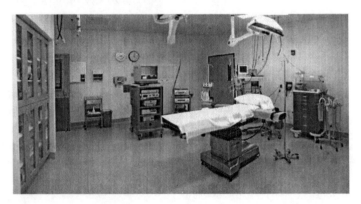

An accredited operating room will have appropriate equipment for any unforeseen event.

HINT: You can save yourself much of this research if you use a surgeon who belongs to ASPS and/or ASAPS because members of these organizations are required to do procedures ONLY in accredited operating rooms.

Additional questions to ask the physician about an in-office OR include:

- *By what agency is the OR accredited?*
  Answer: AAAHC, AAAASF, or JCAHO

- *Who is in charge of the surgical center?*
  Answer: RN or LPN

- *Who will monitor me during surgery?*
  Answer: anesthesiologist or nurse anesthetist

- *Who will monitor me during recovery?*
  Answer: It should be an RN, with the anesthesiologist close by until vitals are normal.

Questions to Ask the Office Staff

- *What is the surgeon's fee for the procedure?*

  Doctors seldom discuss fees. Talk about this with the office manager or accounting person in the doctor's office.

- *Are there additional charges for the operating room? Anesthesia and an anesthesiologist? Any other fees?*

  You should receive, or ask for, an itemization of expected charges. Some of the items to look for are: surgeon's fee, OR fee, anesthesia and anesthesiologist, medication, supplies, garments, and pre-operative testing. Go over it carefully, and don't be afraid to ask if you don't see something or have questions about a particular fee.

- *Is financing available, or can you refer me to a financing program?*

  More and more doctor's offices are making financing available. Usually, it is through a financing company, and the office staff can give you information or a number to call. Sometimes the doctor's office itself will offer payment plans. This is still rare, but don't be afraid to ask. Also, if you have seen several doctors, and the one you really like charges more than the others, ask the office staff about his willingness to come down a bit. It is not unheard of in this very competitive arena. Some offices may also take credit cards, which means you are then financing it through your credit card company.

- *If I do not have the procedure after all, will I be refunded anything I may have paid so far?*

  Different doctors have different policies. If you do pay anything up front, be careful about the approaching procedure date. The closer you get to the date, the stickier it may be to get money back, as with any cancellation. Think about when you book a cruise or a hotel room; you may get a full refund if you cancel 90 days out, but only 75% at 60 days, 50% at 30 days, and so on.

Questions Not to Ask the Doctor

- Do not ask about his personal life, such as dating or family.

- Don't ask how you should get time off work, or whether you should tell your friends you're having cosmetic surgery. These are personal issues, and they're part of the reason you're reading this book first!

- His religious affiliation has nothing to do with his skill as a surgeon.

   One of my clients made it a point to ask if any of the doctors to whom I was referring her were Christian. While I understood and respected that this seemed a valid consideration for her, I stopped her and asked how it would be an advantage for her to seek a Christian doctor. She explained her reasons, and I said I did know of a surgeon who made his Christian affiliation well known.

   Then I showed her a picture of a client who had come to me for help, a former patient of this doctor; the work he had done on her was terrible. My client was shocked. "I'm sure he's a wonderful person and a devout Christian," I said. "But, as you can see, he is not a highly skilled cosmetic surgeon."

   The bottom line is, skill and experience are everything, and personal information doesn't count for much.

As you interview doctors, keep the following important areas in mind. You'll want to find out enough information to do further research, if you want to, before you schedule the operation.

Step 5: Research credentials

Now that you have spoken with at least three doctors, you can take the information you have and do some further research. I suggest you look into the following:

Board certification

   Make sure the surgeon you choose is certified by at least one of the following:

- American Board of Plastic Surgery

- American Board of Otolaryngology (ear, nose, throat—for lipo of the face and neck)

- American Board of Dermatology

Obviously, the type of procedure you want will determine the most appropriate certification for the surgeon you need. Under some circumstances, physicians certified by the American Board of Dermatology perform certain lipo procedures. If a doctor is certified only by one non-cosmetic specialty board, make sure he is qualified and experienced in performing cosmetic surgery. As always, common sense rules—a dermatologist takes care of skin, so he is not necessarily an expert at what's underneath it. For example, one would not go to a dermatologist to have a tummy tuck or nose job.

Red Flag #3: Be aware that board names mean different things. Some so-called "boards" are actually associations that any doctor can join. The American Board of Cosmetic Surgery is one such association. For a surgeon to be truly qualified to perform cosmetic surgery, he must be accredited by an official board of the American Board of Medical Specialties (ABMS). See the back of the book for more information about these boards and certifications.

Hospital privileges

Ask for the names of hospitals where the surgeon has privileges. This information should be on the doctor's CV (resume). Call those hospitals to verify the information. Remember, good hospitals have good doctors on staff. Another way to approach this is to say, "I want to have my procedure done in a hospital; which one would you use?" If the answer is, "No, that's not the way it's done," then he probably doesn't have privileges.

Past problems

By checking with your State Medical Board, you can find out if a surgeon has received any reprimands. What will not show up, of course, are reprimands in any other state. Each state also keeps records of medical malpractice suits filed. How that information can be obtained varies by state. In Georgia, for example, one can call the State Board of Medical Examiners.

General background check

There are Internet-based companies that pull together some of the data for you for a fee. You can search for information on any given surgeon, and what's spit back at you looks basically like the doctor's CV, pared down to information about his medical education and training, licenses and certifications, and disciplinary actions, if any.

One such company, HealthGrades (www.healthgrades .com) does offer a brief free report that is very helpful, and if you do find anything worthy of further investigation, you can buy a more detailed report. Another similar source is Doctor Background Check (www.doctorbackgroundcheck .com), though it does not provide the free general report.

The most comprehensive resource I have found is also the most difficult to get into. The National Practitioner Data Bank (NPDB), a nationwide database of information about doctors, includes hard-to-find data about doctors' track records. Federal law says only certain authorized people can access this information, like hospitals, malpractice attorneys, and health insurance companies. The reason I tell you about this resource that you may never be able to access is that you need to know there may be more detailed information available about a doctor.

Step 6: Assess experience

You want your surgeon to have a good amount of experience in the procedure you want. That does not mean he has to be a veteran. When you go to interview physicians, don't be surprised to meet someone who looks more like an intern on *Scrubs* than the old Marcus Welby, MD! Some of the best cosmetic surgeons today are relatively young, yet highly experienced. How can that be? Well, many have done fellowships specifically in cosmetic surgery. That means that they spent six months to a year doing strictly cosmetic surgery after completing their residency, rather than going directly into practice. This is a concentrated and accelerated way to gain experience in a specific medical field.

Whether young or middle-aged, the fact is that some cosmetic surgeons were at the top of their class, some in the middle, and some closer to the bottom. The important thing to find out about a surgeon's experience is his track record. How many procedures, like the one you want to have, has he performed in the last month? ...in the last year? Is this number on par with the average for others in your area, or cities of similar size? (See the chart on the next page for some national statistics that give you an idea of just how many of each procedure are done.)

Another factor to weigh carefully, along with the facts and figures that illustrate the surgeon's experience, is more esoteric one—talent. Especially in cosmetic surgery, there's an art that goes along with the science of reshaping the body. The cosmetic surgeon has to be a sculptor, in a sense, bringing to the surface a new shape that wasn't there before. This is a subjective area, and I would never suggest that anyone forego any of the stringent credentialing I have harped about so far! It's also not something you'd want to ask your surgeon about. However, if you can readily see it is there, artistic ability or sensibility is a desirable addition to the qualified cosmetic surgeon's little black bag of skills.

Cosmetic Surgery Performed Annually, by Type of Procedure					
Procedure	*2002*	*2003*	*2004*	*2005*	*2006*
Abdominoplasty (tummy tuck)	83,043	117,693	150,987	169,314	172,457
Blepharoplasty (cosmetic eyelid surgery)	229,092	267,627	290,343	231,467	209,999
Botox injection	1,658,667	2,272080	2,837,346	3,294,782	3,181,592
Breast Augmentation	249,641	280,401	334,052	364,610	383,886
Breast Lift	62,458	76,943	98,351	120,980	125,896
Breast Reduction (women)	125,614	147,173	144,374	160,531	145,822
Facelift	124,514	125,581	157,061	150,401	138,245
Forehead lift (brow lift)	65,284	76,696	95,212	71,751	54,149
Gynecomastia, treatment of (male breast reduction)	16,551	22,049	19,636	17,730	23,670
Laser skin resurfacing	72,458	127,470	589,721	475,690	576,509
Lipoplasty (liposuction)	372,831	384,626	478,251	455,489	403,684
Rhinoplasty (nose job)	156,973	172,420	166,187	200,924	141,912

Statistics courtesy of the American Society of Aesthetic Plastic Surgery. Final figures are projected to reflect nationwide statistics and are based on a survey of doctors who have been certified by American Board of Medical Specialties recognized boards, including but not limited to the American Board of Plastic Surgery.

Step 7: Compare pricing

Just as an older surgeon is not necessarily more experienced, a higher-priced surgeon is not necessarily better. Often it is true that a surgeon can demand higher fees because of excellent success rates in the procedures he performs, coupled perhaps with the demographic group to which he caters. If that's so, more power to him! As I mentioned, higher fees for procedures may be based on higher overhead. Just remember, a fancy doctor's office doesn't mean you'll look any better after your surgery. The surgeon's skill and your own participation in the process will determine that.

Remember to inquire about and keep track of the other costs you'll incur on top of the surgeon's fee. These can include:

- Operating room (usually charged by time increments)
- Anesthesiologist or nurse anesthetist
- Anesthetic (general, twilight, and/or local)
- Prescriptions
- Pre-op work (tests, blood work, etc.)
- Garments (for compression after certain procedures)
- Post-op make-up
- Hair removal (example: beard line raised during facelift)
- Home nursing care

Other expenses you may need to consider include:

- Pet care
- Child care
- Transportation to and from doctor's office and/or hospital
- Delivery services (food, courier, etc.)

Step 8: Consider the office staff

Often, the first impression you will have of a doctor comes from his office staff. Are they friendly, helpful, and willing to explain things you want to know? Look for a pleasant phone manner and a general respect in the way they treat patients.

- Do they answer your questions willingly and completely? If they're not very happy to do so at the beginning, think about how you'll feel if you have to call after the surgery with a problem or question.

- Are they prone to talking about other patients in front of you, perhaps even making remarks about how difficult they are? Would you want them talking about you in front of others?

- Are they name-droppers? This shows a lack of confidentiality.

- How do they seem to work together, and what do they say about the surgeon for whom they work? If there is any hint of sniping or backstabbing in the air, it can hinder the efficiency and smooth operation of the practice. Also, the amount of respect for the doctor can be a good indicator of the respect he shows in turn for his staff and his patients.

- Do they have a good attitude? Chances are, you'll be talking to them quite a bit, so you'll want them to be not only cheerful and encouraging, but to have no hang-ups of their own about people having cosmetic surgery—you'll have enough to deal with, thank you very much!

Step 9: Look at before-and-after photos wisely

If you see any such photos of others on whom the doctor has performed the procedure you want, it'll usually be during the interviews with surgeons. There's an art and a science to looking at these photos, and I'm going to reveal all the tricks!

The most important thing to remember is that these pictures are tools that help you envision your own results, but they are not *you*. You will look different—maybe better, maybe not—but different. Also remember that no doctor is going to show you the photos of operations he's not proud of, but don't assume that a doctor with very few before-and-after photos is hiding them because they aren't flattering. It may simply mean he hasn't been in practice long enough to have more or has had patients unwilling to give permission for their pictures to be shown. Keep in mind that it takes years for a doctor to gather before-and-after photos. (Think about whether you would give permission for your before-and-after photos to be used for others to look through.) There may be other reasons the doctor doesn't have photos, too—let me tell you a brief story.

> An excellent young surgeon I know went into practice with an older colleague. They had some differences, and soon it was impossible for them to remain in the same office. The young doctor opened his own office, but due to obstacles and "assignments of property," he had to leave all of his before-and-after photos at the former office. He started all over again—and it had nothing to do with his skill as a surgeon, only with an unfortunate business decision.

When looking at photos, first ask the surgeon whether what you're seeing are actually photos of patients whose operations he has performed. Some cosmetic surgeons use, or supplement their own patient photos with, stock before-and-after pictures. There is nothing really wrong with using stock photos to show you the results of a procedure like yours, but you want to know whether you are looking at that surgeon's handiwork or not.

There are many ways to make someone look good—or ghastly—in a photograph. The average person may not catch that the "after" picture simply shows someone more rested, with make-up on, and/or in better light than the before picture. With my background in modeling and film, I understand acutely how lighting, make-up, head tilt or posture, and distance from the camera can change the way a person looks. In order to pick up the effects of the surgery, rather than these other variables, you'll need to view the photos with an eye for symmetry between the before and after shots. Here are some things to look for. Note how small differences can fool the eye:

- Is the lighting the same? Brighter, more direct light actually makes skin look smoother.

- The pose should be exactly the same in both photos. If it is a headshot, it should be from the same angle, with the chin at the same height. Raising the chin, or thrusting it out, makes the neck look thinner. In a body shot, the limbs should be positioned alike and the posture should be the same. Standing up straighter tightens abdominal muscles, and standing with legs spread differently changes the shape of the hips.

- Does the subject appear to be the same distance from the camera? The closer you get to something, the more imperfections you see.

- Are the photos, in fact, of the same person? This may sound funny, but mix-ups do happen, especially with headless body shots! Try to look for identifying marks like moles or birthmarks that will assure you it is one and the same person. In a torso shot, the belly button can serve as a distinguishing feature. (Forget all that if you're looking at photos of a tummy tuck—for example, after the procedure, a mole can be anywhere from one inch to three inches below where it used to be, and the belly button may look different.)

To test your visual acuity, I've included a set of before-and-after photos on the next page. Can you tell what this person had done? Take a close look and see what you conclude. Was it...

A. liposuction of the abdomen and thighs?

B. liposuction of the abdomen, hips, and buttocks?

C. liposuction of the midriff, abdomen, hips, thighs, and buttocks?

D. none of the above?

(I'll whisper the answer later...on page 91.)

Step 10: Consider Those Red Flags

Let's recap some of the things that should make you stop and think as you go through the meticulous process of choosing your surgeon:

Red Flag #1: If a doctor or his office staff spreads the news about who has been in his office, you need to wonder about the level of confidentiality you'll receive.

Is there name-dropping going on? Instead of impressing you, this should put you on your guard. If they'll talk about someone else's procedure with you, what's to stop them from telling the next patient what surgery you had done?

Before   **After**

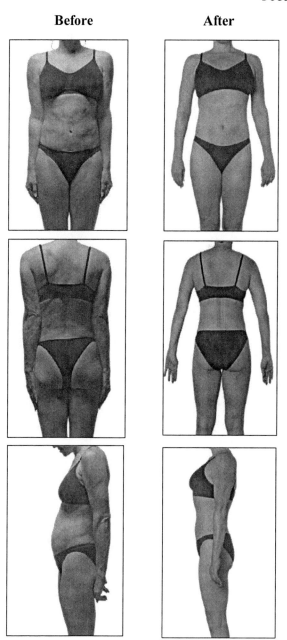

Red Flag #2: If the surgeon doesn't seem to like you asking questions or avoids answering them to your satisfaction, perhaps you need to look for a different surgeon.

As long as your questions pertain to you and your procedure, and the doctor's credentials and experience with it, the doctor should be willing and able to provide the information you need to assess whether you'll book surgery with him or not.

Red Flag #3: Be aware of what boards don't exist or are not recognized by the ABMS (American Board of Medical Specialties). For example, there is an American Board of Cosmetic Surgery, but it is a self-designated board which is not part of ABMS; there is no such thing as Aesthetic Cosmetic Surgery, so don't let anyone try to tell you they hold a certification in it!

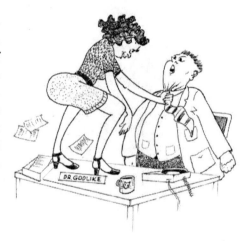

More red flags...

Red Flag #4: Beware of the surgeon who is critical of other doctors.

Does he tell you he's always fixing everybody else's work? Is he condescending when you mention other doctors you're considering? Defensiveness and belittling others can be a sign of professional jealousy or insecurity, and that *may* stem from a less-than-healthy practice.

Red Flag #5: Does the doctor talk more about himself than about you and your procedure?

You want to hire someone to do the best work for you, who will be concerned about you, and who wants to make sure you get what you want, not someone looking at what's in it for him. Remember that arrogance and bravado just might hide a lack of experience and lack of true confidence.

Red Flag #6: When a surgeon shows signs of being abusive to his staff, it may not be long before he turns on you.

If you see a doctor talking down to staff, or even yelling at them, don't walk—run—to the nearest exit. The last thing you need when you're recovering from surgery is a bully telling you what you're doing wrong, and the stage is set for that to be a possibility.

Red Flag #7: The surgeon should advise, caution, and suggest what may be best for you; he should never try to pressure you into something you don't want.

There's a fine line here: you need to listen to the doctor for advice, especially about whether you're a good candidate, and be confident that he is the expert who can make recommendations. But you will probably know when that line is crossed if you feel pushed into considering procedures you're not sure you agree are right, or if he recommends something completely unrelated to the reason you came to see him in the first place. A tell-tale sign you're being led down the wrong path is, "Trust me, I've done *thousands* of these!"

Red Flag #8: After the consultation, does the office staff pester you about booking surgery?

Really, the only time the doctor's office should contact you is if you've shown a real interest in a specific time to schedule surgery.

Red Flag #9: The doctor says, "Don't worry, you look healthy. We don't need to do any kind checkup on you."

Any time you ever have an operation there must always be a health history taken and blood work done before surgery.

Red Flag #10: "Buy one implant now [or one eyelid, or one thigh liposuctioned] and get the other one for free if you book your surgery today!"

You should never feel pressured to book a surgery because of a price break. It's wrong for a doctor's office to give a discount, but you should never be pressured to sign on the dotted line. Buyer beware!

I've found the right doctor! Now what?

You've done your research, talked to people you trust, interviewed doctors, and chosen the best-qualified surgeon for you. Congratulations! So, what comes next?

There are things you will need to discuss with the physician you have picked. Go over your notes, be comfortable about the information you already have, and determine if there are details you need to fill in. The doctor's office should be happy to answer any additional questions before they schedule your liposuction.

Once you schedule, you'll need to be very forthcoming about any medical cautions, drug interactions, lifestyle, and so on. It is vital that you share everything with your surgeon that could in any way affect your surgery. Your doctor is not there to admonish you for smoking or taking a particular drug, but he must be made aware of anything that may affect you medically. It is for your safety.

I know of several patients who had unnecessary complications, and one who actually lost her life, because of not revealing a complete medical history. But I also know of a patient who was totally honest and told his surgeon he was HIV positive, knowing it might disqualify him from having the procedure he wanted. And it may have. However, his particular surgeon decided to do the surgery, and was able to take the precautions that made it safe for everyone involved.

Ok, now for the answer to the before-and-after mystery on page 87. If you answered A, B, or C, look again. The answer is D...this person has had absolutely NO WORK done between the before pictures and after pictures. How is that possible? The differences are in the posture, lighting, and the distance of the subject from the camera. Take a look at how slouching, with chin down, legs together, and arms firmly at sides, produces a dumpy look, while an extended and straight posture reveals a more slender physique. Also notice at how off-center lighting accentuates dimples and furrows, while direct lighting hides them. Get to know these nuances so that you can be an expert at spotting truly excellent surgical work in before-and-after photos!

Choosing the Right Doctor for You:
Doctor Interview Checklist

Make copies of this list and take it along on all your physician interviews. It will help you remember some of the questions to ask. (See pages 68–80 for explanations of these questions.)

☐ How many of my procedure have you performed? (Keep in mind that some procedures are more popular than others.)

☐ Where will the incision be made?

☐ How long will recovery take?

☐ What are the risks involved? What about complications?

☐ Have you personally had any of these (risks, complications) come up? What did you do?

☐ Are there any alternatives to this procedure that you recommend?

☐ If I had to have another operation to correct a complication, would there be another fee?

☐ How would this affect healing time?

☐ Are there any former patients of yours, who have had this procedure, who might be willing to speak with me?

☐ Will you be the surgeon performing the operation?

☐ Will you be available to me after the surgery? (Will you be in town; if not, who will be the doctor on call?) A week later? A month later?

☐ May I see before-and-after photos? Are these your actual patients?

☐ _____

☐ _____

☐ _____

☐ _____

☐ _____

The following questions may be answered on the doctor's CV; check there before you ask these questions at the interview.

☐ Are you Board-certified? By what Board? For how long?

☐ How long have you been performing cosmetic surgery? …this procedure?

☐ What percentage of your current work is cosmetic surgery?

☐ If I decide to have this procedure, where would it be done? Is it an accredited facility?

☐ Can you do my liposuction in a hospital, and if so, which one?

☐ What is your policy concerning confidentiality?

☐ _____

☐ _____

☐ _____

☐ _____

☐ _____

Questions to ask the office staff:

☐ What are the surgeon's fees for this procedure?

☐ Are there additional fees? Do you have an itemized list of what else will be charged?

☐ Does your office have its own, or third-party, financing available or accept credit cards?

☐ If I do not have the procedure, what will I be refunded?

☐ _____

☐ _____

☐ _____

☐ _____

☐ _____

Starting off on the right foot

One of the most important steps in having any cosmetic surgery actually takes place well before the procedure is performed.

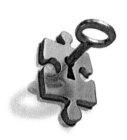

Preparation is key! I can't stress enough that the more you prepare, the better your results can be.

Being well prepared requires that you know what to prepare, and that's what this chapter is all about. In the next few pages, I'll tell you what supplies you'll need to have on hand, how you can let people know what to expect, and what arrangements—made ahead of time—can make your life easier during recovery. As you get ready for your procedure, keep a list of things you learn in this chapter and in the liposuction chapter, as well as the information your surgeon gives you. Then you'll have a handy place to check off that everything is ready.

Here are some important points to start your checklist:

- Follow your doctor's post-op instructions. Believe it or not, having this noted at the top of your list will help you remember to do so in your groggy, sleepy, post-op state!

- Don't do anything your doctor tells you not to do. If, for some reason, you forget and do something you weren't supposed to do, be honest with your doctor and let him know. This is very important.

- If your doctor gives you a sleeping pill to take the night before your procedure, take it. It is very important to get a good night's sleep before your surgery.

- Make sure your air conditioner is running in hot weather and the heat is on in cold weather, so you can come home to a pleasant temperature. Watch the forecast before your surgery, and don't forget to adjust that thermostat if it will be unseasonably warm or cold on the day you'll be coming home after surgery.

- Make sure you have a night light or some form of low wattage light in the bedroom and the bathroom to avoid any accidents in the dark.

- **Things to have on hand:**

  - Anti-bacterial soap or Betadine soap

  - Cotton swabs for cleaning incision sites

  - Peroxide

  - Antibiotic ointment or cream

  - Gauze pads or cotton pads

  - Paper tape (won't pull skin)

- **Transportation:** Make sure you have made arrangements to have reliable transportation home. Check with the doctor's office to see if they provide transportation for patients. Whoever is driving you home should have the following items in the car:

  - A wet washcloth in a zip-locked bag with ice cubes can come in handy if you feel nauseated on your way home. Try placing the cold washcloth on your forehead or neck.

- Have a plastic bag, bowl or trash can (in case of vomiting) in the car on the way home and near your bed at home.

- Place a sunshade on the passenger side car window to block sun and for privacy purposes. Most auto retail shops, like Pep Boys, carry sunshades, as does Toys "R" Us.

Time off

It's better to err on the side of scheduling more time off work than you may need. You can always go back earlier than anticipated and look like a big hero. It's harder to call in later and say you need more time, especially when others may be depending on you to show up on a certain date.

If you work, you'll need to consider at least three important areas: what kind of work you do, how much time you can take, and how it might affect you financially. First and foremost, if you do physically strenuous work, or work outdoors, you may need to request reassignment for several weeks or months depending on the extent of your procedure, beyond just recovery time. Talk to your doctor about the physical requirements of your work and ask for his recommendations.

Many people who work for companies have two weeks per year vacation time. After some procedures, this may not be long enough. One option might be to request additional unpaid time, or sick leave, or personal days—whatever your company will allow. Others, such as entrepreneurs and commissioned sales people, have income based on the work they actually do, so if they aren't working, nothing is coming in. In this case, there may be more flexibility about time taken off, but you'll need to add living expenses during downtime to what you'll pay for surgery.

Each person's healing process is unique, but there are some average durations that parts of the healing process involve to help you plan. Also talk to your doctor and consider his recommendations in your specific case.

One thing that can give you more time off is scheduling the procedure before a holiday. The tradeoff is that you won't get to go to that big July 4th picnic, or join the family at Thanksgiving, but many people find this an easy way to have more recovery time. Below is a rundown of major holidays that most companies in the United States observe. If you are planning to have your surgery around Thanksgiving, Christmas, or New Year's, you'll need to book it far in advance. It's one of the most popular times for surgery. Also find out if there are additional "no business" days planned for your company in a particular year. And, although it's not an official holiday, you may get some additional time to yourself if you have kids who are planning a spring break trip.

Holidays	
JANUARY	New Year's Day
	Martin Luther King Jr. Birthday
FEBRUARY	President's Day
APRIL	Passover
	Good Friday / Easter
MAY	Memorial Day
JULY	Independence Day
SEPTEMBER	Labor Day
	Rosh Hashanah*
	Yom Kippur*
OCTOBER	Columbus Day
NOVEMBER	Thanksgiving
DECEMBER	Christmas
	Chanukah

September or October

Preparing the people in your life

Aside from preparing the most important person—YOU!—preparing your family and others close to you is also vital.

People you must tell you are having surgery

- You need to tell at least one person that you are having surgery.

  Someone will need to bring you home after your procedure and stay with you for at least the first day and night. If there is no one who can do this, there are nurses and sitters you can hire. Some cities also have recovery centers. Check the Yellow Pages or the Internet for resources in your area, such as nursing services.

- Your spouse or significant other

  Every once in a while I will have a client (and this goes for both men and women) who thinks he or she can go through cosmetic surgery without telling a spouse or significant other. Forget it, get it out of your head, it cannot happen. The reason is that you're being put to sleep and having an operation; if it were a different type of surgery—like having your gall bladder removed—you would certainly tell him or her, and this should be no different.

  Spouses or significant others sometimes are supportive of your decision, and sometimes they are not. What you must keep in mind is that you're doing this for you and not for anyone else. But, if it's causing a knockdown drag-out fight every time the subject is brought up, then you need to get rid of the jerk or maybe seek some counseling to get to the bottom of what's really going on with the other person. Sometimes what's going on can be the following:

- They've heard a horror story about cosmetic surgery and they are fearful for you. If you find out that's what it is, tell them they should speak to the doctor or go on a consultation with you to get reassurance.

- They're afraid that you are going to look better and be more attractive to other people. This is jealousy, and it is definitely *their* problem, and they need to work on that issue through professional counseling.

- They've known someone that has died under anesthesia. In this case, they need to speak to the anesthesiologist for reassurance.

- Perhaps they can't stand that you are spending money on yourself!

- Roommate

  Basically, whoever you live with will need to know what you'll be going through. You'll want to make arrangements ahead of time regarding housework, taking out the trash, and all the daily tasks you normally share. Also make your roommate aware that you need peace and quiet while you're recovering.

- Parents (if you're close to them, or perhaps aren't married or in a relationship)

To tell or not to tell

Some people who you may not want to tell about your procure include the following:

- Anyone with a big mouth.

  This applies only if you don't want others to know you're having cosmetic surgery.

- Anyone who might try to use it against you in the future.

  Only you know if there is anyone out there who doesn't wish you all the best. This can include a jealous ex, a competitive colleague, or competition in general if you are in a high-profile field.

Now, you need to decide for yourself whether to tell the following people or not.

Children

No one knows your children better than you, but I think it's always a good idea to prepare them as much as possible for

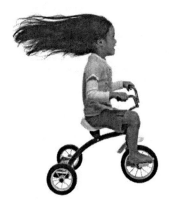

what they might see once you come out of surgery, unless you plan to be away from them during your healing period.

If you have small children, hyper children, or very demanding children, you will need to be separated from them (meaning no physical contact) for at least the first 72 hours, depending on your procedure. The last thing you want, especially if you have had liposuction or a tummy tuck, is your child body-slamming you.

First, you should consider having young children go on vacation, or to camp, or to grandma's house for at least a week. If that is not possible, it is important that you tell your children you are going to have surgery and that you are going to be OK. If your kids will be at home and you are the "taxi mom" (or dad), plan ahead for who will pick up the kids from school, how they will get to Scouts or sport practices, and so on.

Children become very scared when they see their parents looking bruised and battered. Showing them photographs of what you may possibly look like can help ease their fears beforehand (you may be able to get photos from your doctor). If you have had any breast surgery or a tummy tuck along with your liposuction, which limit you physically for a few weeks, be sure to tell your children that you will not be able to lift anything for a few weeks, including them.

Remember, if you are a parent, this is your time to do something for you. You may want to have a sit-down talk with your children to help them understand. The more prepared everyone is, the better it is for you, the healing patient. If one of your concerns is not having too many people know what you are having done, it is important to tell your children during this conversation that they cannot tell other people. If you have a child who cannot help telling the neighbors everything (also known as diarrhea of the mouth!), you might consider sending him or her to camp or grandma's, and forget discussing the procedure.

My experience in the past with young children has been that, when the whole surgical experience is downplayed, children hardly even notice, or they find it amusing.

Teenagers

Teenagers will be, well...teenagers. What you don't need is someone making fun of you or criticizing you. Teenagers have a tendency to do this to their parents.

As far as teenagers go, it's pretty black and white—they're either for it or against it, and they'll let you know. But what you don't need is a teenager giving you a hard time about your decision. If you anticipate a possible negative reaction from a child, you may decide to have surgery while they are away at camp or with the grandparents, or you pack your bag and go somewhere else. Being in a positive atmosphere is very important during a healing period.

Please keep in mind that this is for you, and you don't need approval from anyone but yourself. It's a good idea to sit down with your teenagers and tell them that you don't need any criticism or harassment from them during this time. What you do need is to rest and recover as soon as possible. A week to ten-day separation from your children is highly recommended if possible. However, only you know your children and how they might react.

Pets

Those of you who have pets—whether cats or dogs, a horse, or a pig (yes, I know someone who has a potbellied pig in the house)—you know they require care. As much as you love having them around, you don't need to be stressing out about whether your animals have enough food or water or have been out enough

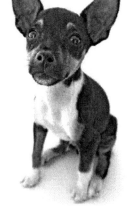

times. If your cat or dog sleeps with you, guess what: they're not going to be sleeping with you while you are recovering. You need to have your environment as clean as possible, and definitely not be pounced on when a little four-legged beast feels like playing.

I have a beautiful little dog myself. But he is a handful (I admit it; I've spoiled him rotten!). During my past procedures, I always made arrangements for someone to take care of him outside my home. Trust me, it's the best way to make sure you get the rest and recovery time you need. And your pets won't be confused by you being grouchy and unable to play with them.

Preparing your home

Make a list of couriers that can deliver supplies, medication, food, and other items, or a good friend or family member for backup. Have a list of restaurants in the area that deliver—but be sure you know their food is what you'll need to eat (not too spicy or full of sodium).

Many clients have told me that they just don't know what to do with themselves while recovering at home. You might want to stock up on

- magazines
- books
- books-on-tape
- movies
- puzzles

It could be a good time to take up or rekindle a hobby, such as

- knitting

- playing cards

- playing video games (handheld)

- listening to a talk radio

- updating your palm pilot or address book

- putting together a photo album, assembling a scrapbook, or organizing your recipes

- making a tape or burning a CD of your favorite songs, or downloading new songs to your MP3 player or iPod

Have your bed freshly made and your room prepared for arrival after surgery, with extra pillows to prop up on. If your bed is upstairs, you may want to relocate it or pick a different place to recover—stairs can be a bear after some procedures.

Food

What you eat will be one of the most important factors for swift healing. Have an adequate supply of healthy food and prepared meals that are **low in sodium and not spicy**. Be sure you have enough on hand for at least the time you will be homebound. Prepare some meals ahead of time, because you won't want to fix anything after your surgery. Remember to keep your **diet high in protein** after surgery to heal faster.

More about salt and sodium

Should you avoid salt like the plague? According to Carolyn O'Neil, dietitian and author of *The Dish on Eating Healthy and Being Fabulous!*, the answer is no…salt is not taboo. Table salt is 40% sodium (the other 60% is chloride), an important nutrient that balances the body's fluids and helps muscles and nerves do their work. Adding table salt to foods is a major source of our daily sodium.

However, we also get sodium in many other ways. The added table salt often takes sodium levels over the top. The U.S. Dietary Guidelines recommend that healthy adults consume no more than 2300 milligrams of sodium per day. That's about a teaspoon of salt…if you didn't get sodium any other way. But most people don't realize all the sodium they are getting in other ways and consume around 4000 milligrams a day! The good news is that studies show that when we cut back on salt, out taste buds adjust.

When you are covering from a procedure, you need to watch your sodium intake because it can affect how much you swell and how fast you heal.

- Read labels. Look for the number of milligrams of sodium included in foods.

- Many canned or processed foods like pickles, gravies, salad dressings, barbecue and other sauces, soups, soy sauce, and broths are usually high in sodium. Avoid processed foods during recovery.

- Cheese and smoked meats contain high amounts of sodium. Use these in moderation.

Instead of consuming foods high in salt, try these alternatives:

- Eat more fruits and vegetables. They're naturally low in sodium. In addition, they are high in potassium, which acts as a counter-balance to sodium. They can help regulate the fluids that cause swelling.

- Remember to drink lots of water; the more you drink, the more fluids you will flush out of your system.

- Grapefruit and cranberry juices are natural diuretics. When you're tired of water or crave a cocktail (and you know you shouldn't have alcohol while recovering!), try a "mocktail" made of juices and club soda. Experiment to find the flavors you like.

Dealing with nausea

One of the typical results of surgery—usually related to the anesthesia and some of the pain medications used—is nausea. As you know, having an operation requires that your stomach be empty, and that sets the stage for your body to react to the drugs, making you nauseated. There are some things you can do before, during, and after surgery to help prevent or relieve nausea.

First, avoid alcohol, caffeine, and rich foods before an operation. Of course, you will stop all food and beverage intake the night before, but you should avoid these items for 24 to 48 hours beforehand. If you smoke, you should quit at least two weeks prior to surgery; besides being very detrimental to healing because it obstructs oxygen flow, smoking may contribute to nausea as well, perhaps due to the carbon monoxide it brings into the body.

If you have a history of nausea from anesthesia, are prone to motion sickness, or are simply afraid you will get sick, ask your anesthesiologist or nurse anesthetist to administer anti-nausea drugs before and during the operation.

After surgery, continue to avoid caffeine, alcohol, nicotine, and rich foods. Also avoid making quick movements, as this can make you dizzy and result in nausea. If you do feel nauseated, here are some things you can try (as always, check with your doctor about anything you plan to use):

- Acupressure wristbands (like Sea-Bands)—these bands go on both wrists and provide acupressure to the main artery in your wrist. I have used these both when having surgery and on boats, and they really work! They can even be worn into surgery.

- Nausea patches—these administer small doses of anti-nausea drugs; they are available by prescription only. These also can be worn into surgery.

- Dramamine—an over-the-counter motion sickness drug.

- Ginger root—ginger is a natural remedy used for thousands of years. To lessen nausea, you can chew raw or candied ginger root or drink ginger ale or ginger tea; it can also be found in pill form (as always, check with your doctor before taking anything, especially because ginger can also prevent blood clotting). One study even showed ginger more effective than Dramamine. Ginger has been found to have many pain-relieving compounds and anti-cramping compounds, and the active ingredient for nausea prevention seems to be *gingerol*, a type of *oleoresin* (a combination of phenylalkylketones and aromatic oils). It also has over a dozen antioxidants that may also help bring down swelling.

Prescriptions

Make sure you have all **prescriptions filled before surgery**. Also be sure to read on your pill bottle whether you are able to get refills or not. Have the phone number of a drug store that will deliver. You don't want to run out of a prescription when you most need it and are least able to go out and get it! If there aren't any drugstores that deliver in your area, have a friend get your refill or call a courier service. Also have your doctor's number handy, in case you have questions or need to have him call in a prescription or refill for you. Have the pharmacy's number handy to give to your doctor.

If you're given prescriptions for controlled substances, such as narcotics (like Demerol), be aware that the doctor cannot phone in the prescription for that—a written prescription will need to be hand-delivered to the drugstore. You, or the person who will be taking you home, will need to pick it up and take it to the drug store. You'll want to make sure ahead of time that it's OK if someone other than you picks up such a prescription. (I know it sounds funny, but if the person picking up your prescription has had a drug problem in the past, you might want to count your pills when they arrive!)

If you need a refill, don't wait until 4:55 p.m. on a Friday afternoon to call it in. Get your refills taken care of well before the weekend.

SUN	MON	TUES	WED	THUR	FRI	SAT
SUN MORN 7AM-9AM	MON MORN 7AM-9AM	TUES MORN 7AM-9AM	WED MORN 7AM-9AM	THUR MORN 7AM-9AM	FRI MORN 7AM-9AM	SAT MORN 7AM-9AM
SUN NOON 11AM-1PM	MON NOON 11AM-1PM	TUES NOON 11AM-1PM	WED NOON 11AM-1PM	THUR NOON 11AM-1PM	FRI NOON 11AM-1PM	SAT NOON 11AM-1PM
SUN EVE 4PM-6PM	MON EVE 4PM-6PM	TUES EVE 4PM-6PM	WED EVE 4PM-6PM	THUR EVE 4PM-6PM	FRI EVE 4PM-6PM	SAT EVE 4PM-6PM
SUN BED 8PM-10PM	MON BED 8PM-10PM	TUES BED 8PM-10PM	WED BED 8PM-10PM	THUR BED 8PM-10PM	FRI BED 8PM-10PM	SAT BED 8PM-10PM

It is not unusual for patients to get confused after surgery. After having my liposuction, I took a pain pill and five minutes later couldn't remember if I'd taken it! A great way to avoid this madness is to get a **pill organizer** before you have your procedure, one that has days of the week and times of day. Or use little Dixie cups and write the days and times on them. Then put your pills in the slots that match when you're supposed to take the pills. I suggest doing this several days in advance.

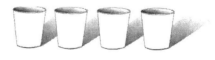

Keep in mind that some drugs (including over-the-counter meds and even some supplements) shouldn't be taken together. Your doctor may go over drug interactions with you, but if he doesn't, be sure to read all the labels and talk to the pharmacist when you get your prescriptions filled.

Weight

If you have any weight to lose, do so prior to surgery. Losing weight affects the elasticity of the skin, and if you do it after liposuction, you might end up with new sags! This includes losing weight before facial surgery.

Sleep

Some people experience problems sleeping after surgery. Sometimes, this is simply due to sleeping all day after anesthesia, and your internal clock is all mixed up. Sometimes it's a side effect of pain pills. Sometimes it's an after-effect of the anesthesia itself. Some surgeons will prescribe sleeping pills and others will not. What's sure is that when you don't sleep, you're not getting the rest you need to heal as well as possible. If your doctor recommends you not take sleeping pills, don't.

Try other sleep aids, like Benadryl or Tylenol PM. These are over-the-counter medications, but they can also leave you groggy and result in something that feels like a hangover. There are also natural remedies, like herbal teas or melatonin[3] (which doesn't work for everyone). However, if you are taking drugs that you've had prescribed after surgery, you need to ask about interactions with anything else you take. Whatever you decide you'd like to try, ASK YOUR DOCTOR before taking it.

---

3 **melatonin:** naturally occurring hormone associated with sleep; synthetic forms of melatonin are sold as sleep aids

After liposuction of the face or breast, you will need to **sleep on your back**. For some people, this is difficult, as they usually sleep on their side or stomach. I've had some clients flip out about sleeping on their back more than they do about having an operation! Here are some tips to make it easier:

- Start training yourself to sleep on your back prior to the procedure.

- Make sure a pillow is always under your knees to reduce stress on your lower back.

- Try sleeping on the sofa.

- A recliner is fine after facial surgery, but not for a tummy tuck or lipo of the stomach area (because you can't use abdominal muscles to get up out of it).

- If you have an outdoor lounge chair, try bringing it into the house and sleeping on that.

Some people find it easier and more comfortable to sleep in a reclining chair, or a chaise lounger with a thick comfy pad (remember to keep your head above your heart if you have had lipo of the face or neck). One of my clients even had one of those electric beds that you can raise the head and feet! But you can use your own bed, and add comfort by using a foam egg crate and a bunch of pillows. I recommend **seven pillows**—two or three under the head and 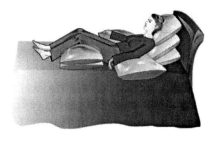 upper back, one under each elbow, and one to two under the knees. And we're not talking thin squishy pillows that smash down—make sure pillows are medium firm.

If you're traveling for your procedure

If you need to or decide to go out of town to have surgery, you should spend at least the first phase of your recovery there. Count on at least a few days and up to three weeks, depending on the procedure. There are some things you'll want to do ahead of time to make your recovery away from home more comfortable.

Of course, you'll talk to your surgeon and his staff about your stay. Find out if they have a special deal set up with any hotels in the area. Some surgeons actually have or are associated with special surgery recovery centers, but this is still rare.

To avoid blood clots, plan to arrive at least 24 hours before your procedure, and don't plan to fly back home until 3 to 5 days after the procedure (or until you are fully able to walk after lower body lipo).

If possible, you'll want to stay in a **suite with a kitchenette**. There are things you will be eating and drinking that room service won't have. Request a no-smoking room, and be sure it's in a quiet area. You might even ask to stay in a room designed for people with disabilities—the showers are easier to get in and out of, with seats and handrails in them.

For all procedures, you'll need to have someone with you for at least the first day and night, sometimes longer. Be sure to make arrangements for this with the hotel. If you can't bring a friend or family member on the trip, make arrangements for a visiting nurse (ask your surgeon's office for recommendations or contact a medical staffing agency).

You'll want to check in and set up your room for recovery prior to your operation. That means letting the hotel know about your needs and making sure no maids come in and change things! You will also need to tell the hotel that you may checking out and back in; confirm ahead of time that you can do this.

If you check out (and will be checking back in after surgery), and you need to pack up all your stuff during that time, you'll need someone to help you set up the room and unpack your things when you check in again. You *will not* be able to do it yourself! See if you can hire a helper through the hotel, or ask the visiting nurse service you'll be using if the nurse can help you with this (sometimes they are not allowed to). Be sure to make these arrangements ahead of time.

Before leaving home, you'll want to ship certain items to your hotel. You won't want to take it all on the plane and, remember, you need to limit your lifting after surgery. Make sure they will arrive a day or two before you do, and ask the hotel to hold the package until you get there. You will have a personal list of what to bring, of course, but here are some items you'll want to think about having:

- Staple foods that room service won't have, including
  - Protein drinks or powders
  - Favorite cereals; small pasta
  - Coffee, tea; favorite sweetener and creamer
- A good carving knife
- Sippy cup
- Insulated cup
- Bendable long straws
- Hand blender
- Laundry detergent and dryer sheets; quarters for the washer and dryer (having the hotel do laundry is expensive—you or your companion can do it for much

less; remember, don't ship a whole box of detergent—
you'll just need a baggy full or so)

- Comfort items:
  - Personal sheets and favorite pillow (remember to request extra pillows at the hotel to prop up in bed)
  - Wedge pillow
  - Slip-on shoes
  - Robe and slippers
  - Favorite stuffed animal
  - Photos of family, friends, and pets (to make it feel more like home)
  - Feel-good shower items (soaps, lotions)— remember, no tub baths until your incisions are completely healed
  - Meditation tapes
  - Sound machine (white noise) to block out hotel noises and help you sleep
- Pill organizer (with days of week and times of day)
- Any medications you need to take (for cholesterol, thyroid, heart, etc.)
- Night lights (take an extra one as backup)
- Shipping tape and premade labels for sending back packages
- Things to do while recovering (think about things that you never have time for or that would normally bore you out of your mind):
  - Magazines, books, tapes, videos, puzzles, crosswords, drawing pad and pencils, books on tape, PlayStation, Xbox

- Projects like photo albums, scrapbooks, updating of address book, holiday card list, knitting, needlepoint, stationery to catch up on correspondence, inputting data into a database

- Scissors to cut open packages, prepare entries for scrapbook, trim gauze bandages, etc.

- Tape—both surgical and transparent

- Notepads, sticky notes (the sticky notes come in handy for reminders on the medications you'll be taking, as well as being great bookmarks for anything you're reading)

Also make sure to tell the hotel that **housekeeping should NOT throw away the box** that your things arrived in! You'll need it to ship them back home. Also find out whether you can arrange for the hotel to ship a package back, or make direct arrangements with a shipping company like UPS, FedEx, DHL, etc.

When you repack to send the package home, put as much in it as you can so you have lighter luggage to take with you on the plane. Don't forget to pack all sharp objects (carving knife, scissors) in the package to be shipped, or they'll be confiscated at the airport!

Other things to ask the hotel:

- Do they have a business center where you can send and check email? Some people prefer to bring their own laptop, in which case you should ask if you can connect in your room and if they offer high speed Internet access. But remember, a laptop is a heavier item to be carrying on the plane, especially when you may not be able to carry much after surgery. If you are comfortable shipping it, that's another option.

- Is there a VCR or DVD player or a PlayStation or Xbox in the room or available for rental? Can you rent videos? Most hotels offer pay-per-view movies, of course, but remember you'll be on medication and it may take you several tries to get through a film without falling asleep— and you don't want to pay for it over and over! If there is no VCR or DVD player in the room, ask to speak with the hotel engineer to see if one can be connected to the TV in the room—for some, you may need a converter, and you'll need to know what kind. Also remember that you can bring your laptop or a portable DVD player.

- Is there a radio? CD player? Tape player?

- Is there a safe for valuables?

- Do they cash travelers' checks? Personal checks? Don't assume they do; many hotels actually do not.

- Do they have—or can the concierge arrange—services such as massage, manicure/pedicure, reflexology, hair salon services? All of these things can help you feel great before your trip back home.

- Is there a courier service (and what are the fees) in case you need food, medications, or anything else delivered to you?

Be sure to have extra checks with you for unforeseen expenses, as well a credit card for restaurant deliveries, courier fees, medication (and make sure there's a drugstore nearby), personal services, and other things you may need to buy while there.

Be sure to arrange transportation to and from the airport on both ends, and to and from the doctor's office in between. For the return trip, arrange with the airline to have a wheelchair ready for you. Even if you feel you don't need it, trust me, it'll make things much easier and safer for you—you shouldn't underestimate risks like getting weak in the airport, not making a connecting flight because you can't move fast, and so on.

Also check into whether the person picking you up back home can have a pass to meet you at the gate (this varies by airline and airport)—and be sure to find out *exactly* where he or she needs to go to pick up that pass on the day you arrive.

Pre-op procedures

Usually about two weeks prior to surgery, you'll have some tests and paperwork to do. Depending on your age, the routine will be something like this:

Under 40 years old	Over 40	Over 50
Blood work	Blood work	Blood work
	Chest x-ray	Chest x-ray
	EKG (maybe)	EKG

Pre-op tests will be ordered for you based on your medical history and initial physical exam. Certain routine tests that should be done (better safe than sorry) before elective surgery include:

Urinalysis is routine and may point up any renal or urinary tract problems, especially in older patients.

Blood tests, including a complete blood count (cbc); clotting studies may be done if you take certain drugs or have bleeding tendencies.

A chest x-ray may be done if you smoke or have respiratory problems. For men over 40 and women over 45, or anyone with a history of cardiac problems, an **electrocardiograph** (EKG) should be performed.

Other tests may be performed either routinely or based on your specific case. They may include **pulmonary** (lung) function studies and **blood chemistries**. **HIV** testing is not routine, but has far-reaching implications both medically and legally. If you have not been tested, you may be requested to have this test, which cannot be performed without your explicit consent.

Fat be gone!
Liposuction and what it can do

Liposuction is one of the most popular cosmetic surgery procedures performed today. Known medically as suction lipectomy or lipoplasty, it refers to the removal of fat, or lipids, from between skin and muscle.

In the early 1980s, the French technique for suction-assisted lipectomy (SAL) revolutionized the ability to re-contour the body. In the hands of properly trained and experienced surgeons, the procedure is very safe today and more effective than previous, cruder approaches. In less than a decade, suction lipectomy became the most commonly performed cosmetic surgery procedure in America; in 2006, cosmetic surgeons performed more than 400,000 procedures to remove unwanted fat from various areas of the body. Nearly 12 percent of these operations were performed on men.

"The big change since the inception of liposuction is that it is a much safer technique," comments Dr. James Wells, a surgeon in Long Beach, CA. "The quality of the equipment is much better, we have more options, instrument designs, new power-assisted devices, and newer ultrasonic devices. We know more about the physiology of liposuction and the bruising. When we first started doing it, the concept of tumescent fluid was not there—tumescent allows a higher margin of safety, allows easier removal of fat with less bleeding and bruising, and allows some of the liposuction procedures to be done with the local anesthesia in the tumescent solution. It does require that the physician be aware of the amount of local anesthetic being given to a patient over a short period of time, however, to avoid lidocaine toxicity and an unwanted drug reaction."

Liposuction can be used pretty much head to toe. Performed properly on a good candidate, liposuction removes fatty bulges and leaves little scarring. It is *not* a diet aid, but rather works best for fit individuals who have localized deposits of fat that just won't go away with exercise. It helps to contour the body and can help with such problems as a "double chin" or "weak chin," in which a chin implant can make the jaw line more prominent while liposuction reduces fat deposits under the chin and in the jowls. Popular areas for lipo include upper arms, "love handles" along the back and hips, stomach, inner and outer thighs, upper arms, and chest (for reduction in men; it is also beginning to be used in female breast reduction).

With the advent of "liposculpture" (also called selective, precision, or fine- or micro-liposuction), other areas previously considered off-limits are being targeted for small-volume contouring. This includes the neck and face where there is less fat, upper back and around the spine, calves, knees, and ankles.

Liposuction is often an "add-on" to other operations. It is not uncommon for a patient to have liposuction of the abdomen or thighs while also having surgery on the eyes, nose, breasts, and so on. It also often assists in achieving the full effect of a procedure like a tummy tuck or facelift.

No two persons, despite similar appearances, will respond to lipo in exactly the same way. In addition to the skill and experience of the surgeon, the final result depends on such factors as the following:

- tobacco, alcohol, and drug use
- overall health
- underlying bone structure and musculature
- skin condition
- amount and location of fat

The way to see whether you are a good candidate is to find a qualified surgeon and have him evaluate your specific situation.

Some people who think they want liposuction actually find out that sagging muscles, not fat, are causing their potbelly. Or, they may be told their skin is not elastic enough to "bounce back" after the procedure and additional work would be needed to achieve the results they want. It is the doctor's responsibility to assess the area where you want liposuction, explain to you what the problem actually is, and then suggest the best course of treatment.

Remember that, with liposuction, it is better to suction a conservative amount of fat. You can always do more later. You don't want to end up with dimpling or indentations by trying to take out too much. If too much is removed, there is now a way to replace some of the fat, but it is a long, tedious, and very expensive procedure.

Sometimes people who are overweight in general will look at liposuction as a way to remove a large volume of fat at once. While this can have dramatic results, there are higher risks involved. The patient is under sedation longer, larger amounts of fluids are needed, and blood transfusion may be required. A good doctor will recommend that any large-volume liposuction procedure be done in the hospital due to the precautionary measures available there.

There are different terms you will hear in connection with liposuction today. I'll mention the major ones here, but note that there are variations on these:

Tumescent Lipoplasty is a method of preparation that is used to assist liposuction techniques. It involves injecting the areas for liposuction with a saline solution containing lidocaine with adrenaline, used for local anesthesia as well as to reduce the bleeding or bruising. It also contains a bicarbonate solution which neutralizes some of pain associated with injection of the tumescent solution.

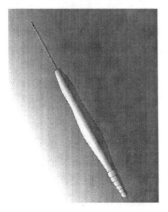

*The instrument used in liposuction is called a **cannula**. It is similar in circumference to a pencil and is made of hollow stainless steal. Inserted into the incision, the cannula sucks fat into a receptacle. The removed fat is measured in liters or cubic centimeters (CCs).*

The **Super-Wet Method** is similar to tumescent but, contrary to the name, less fluid is injected. The amount of fluid used typically equals the amount of fat removed, but there is a bit more blood loss. The advantage is that the Super-Wet Method takes about one fourth the time to perform (depending on the area being liposuctioned) and, since there is less chance of too much fluid being pumped into the body, Super-Wet is generally safer than tumescent.

Mesotherapy is a technique (invented by Dr. Michel Pistor in 1952) in which medication is injected into the mesoderm, the layer of fat and connective tissue under the skin. It has been used for weight loss, cellulite reduction, hair loss, and corrections of scarring and lumpiness following liposuction. But the formulas vary widely and there is no standardized injection protocol; this prompted the American Society for Aesthetic Plastic Surgery (ASAPS) in May 2007 to issue "a warning against the use of injection fat loss treatments. Patients are advised to avoid these procedures, which are commonly known as lipolysis, mesotherapy, or the brand names Lipodissolve and Lipostabil." Then, in September 2007, the FDA approved a clinical trial investigating the safety and efficacy of one type of injection lipolysis treatment. The study, designed and funded by The Aesthetic Surgery Education and Research Foundation (ASERF) with FDA supervision, follows patients for 46 weeks to who receive one form of injection. At the time of this printing, this trial was just beginning. So, if you are interested in this technique, make sure you find out the latest results of this and other possible trials.

Ultrasound-Assisted Lipoplasty (UAL)—This technique has been used in Europe for quite some time and was introduced in the United States in the mid-1990s. This procedure also utilizes the cannula, but it is slightly different and connected to an ultrasound generator. The sound waves help break down the fat and may be able (in some areas) to remove more fat than the tumescent method. It works best on "love handles," upper abdomen, back, and chest (for men). Some doctors, though not all, believe that skin retracts better after ultrasonic lipoplasty than after the tumescent method. It is significantly more expensive than tumescent and, as with any surgery, there are risks that can include the following:

- Time spent in surgery is longer.

- A few patients may experience a permanent burning sensation in the areas that were liposuctioned.

- There is a very slight risk of skin burn from the inside out.

- A pocket of fluid that collects under the skin—called a seroma—can sometimes occur, which the doctor must then drain.

Power-Assisted Lipoplasty (PAL)—This form of liposuction uses a reciprocating cannula (one whose tip moves back and forth very quickly). As this cannula moves through tissue more easily, many doctors believe that this method cuts down on surgery duration and healing time.

"The introduction of ultrasonic and power-assisted equipment has made a big difference because we can remove the fat in a much easier fashion," Dr. Wells describes. "Newer cannulas are smaller and less apt to create injury but still require a skilled physician experienced in the use of the equipment. Liposuction has come a long way. Most recently, we've had other ultrasonic, sound-wave formats, and the cannulas are even smaller. In addition, there's pulsed energy now, which seems to more efficiently break down the fat and extract it. It's another generation of equipment."

Liposuction can be used to remove unwanted fat from a wide array of body areas. It is ideal for the removal of stubborn fat deposits that you just can't seem to exercise away in areas including:

- chin and jowls (through liposuction alone or in conjunction with a facelift)
- upper arms
- above the breast
- breast (there is a liposuction-assisted breast reduction procedure)
- chest (for men)
- upper abdomen
- lower abdomen
- waist
- flank (lower back)
- buttocks
- hips and thighs
- knees, calves, and ankles

Light-Based Liposuction—Another option for small pockets of fat is **laser-assisted liposuction** (also called SmartLipo), which uses a laser to heat up and liquefy fat cells, making it easier to remove the fat with suction. According to Chicago plastic surgeon Dr. Talmage Raine, "Laser liposuction, like any form of liposuction, can be used to reduce the circumference of the thigh by several inches." This procedure is performed with local anesthesia and a cannula that's smaller than those used in other lipo methods. Depending on the area treated, incisions can be so small that they don't even require a stitch, which also means smaller scars. As an added benefit, the laser helps tighten overlying skin. And because the laser seals off blood vessels, there is less bleeding, swelling, and bruising, resulting in quicker recovery. Patients can be back to work in a couple of days. Pain is minimal, but Dr. Raine says, "Patients may feel a little sore." Though not a substitute for conventional liposuction, SmartLipo is ideal for small areas of stubborn fat, such as those on the face, neck, arms, and abdomen.

Liposuction does not replace weight loss. I can't emphasize enough that, if you are dieting, wait until after you have reached your goal and maintained your weight for a substantial amount of time—I say at least one year. Your weight must be stable so that you don't gain it back through the remaining fat cells expanding.

Rumor has it that, once an area has been liposuctioned, you can't gain weight there. This is false! Remember, not every fat cell is removed (they can't all be). If you yo-yo in weight and have liposuction in your low-weight cycle, and then gain 10 pounds or more, don't be surprised if that area gets lumpy, bumpy, and wavy. Not a pretty sight. And you can't blame your doctor—he didn't make you stuff your face.

Now, this is very important if you want good results: If you have lost a significant amount of weight (40 pounds or more), you need to tell the doctor this, as this affects the elasticity of the skin.

What results can be expected?

As with any procedure, the best results can be expected for ideal patients, and with liposuction the ideal is someone who is relatively young while skin is still elasctic (40 or younger is best—after 40, or if you have stretch marks, it may be difficult to predict skin elasticity after lipo), physcially fit, and with small concentrations of fat to be removed. Remember that this is a shaping procedure, not a weight loss solution!

Results can vary, as you'll read below, but basically depend on the volume of fat in relationship to the skin surface. If the skin recoils, like a balloon deflating, results will be smooth. If it gathers, though, like a thicker beach ball that's lost air, there could be an irregular result. Your surgeon can explain more about expected results for your particular case, but here are a few general experiences.

Chin and jowls: Many people, male and female, have had great results with the removal of concentrated fat under the chin. This can create a tighter, more youthful profile. Sometimes the doctor will recommend a chin implant to further enhance that contour if you have a weak chin.

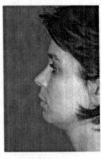 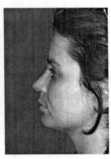

Liposuction with chin implant.

(Photos courtesy of Dr. Mark Beaty, Alpharetta, GA)

Before   *After*

Sometimes, the doctor may find that the problem is actually muscles that need tightening, and liposuction may be used as an adjunct. Liposuction also can be very useful in removing excess fat in the jowls and chin during a facelift, making the face thinner as well as tighter during this procedure.

Liposuction of the upper arm.

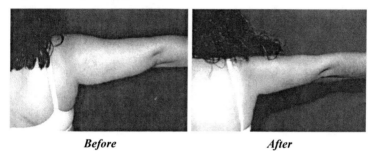

Before   **After**

Treatment of gynecomastia, also known as male breast reduction.

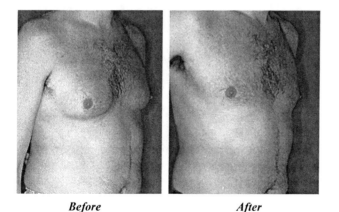

Before   **After**

Upper body: Fat in the upper arms—the kind that wiggles when a person waves—is a typical upper body liposuction target. The technique is also used in conjunction with breast reduction to remove adjoining fat from the armpits and sides. Some surgeons are also beginning to use liposuction on the breast itself, creating a new "scarless breast lift." (Don't get too excited, girls—it is limited in this use.)

Before   *After*

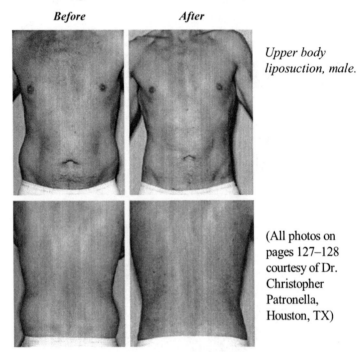

Upper body liposuction, male.

(All photos on pages 127–128 courtesy of Dr. Christopher Patronella, Houston, TX)

Lower body: Liposuction does not improve dimpled skin or cellulite. This dimpling actually happens in the layer above the fat, and liposuction in an area where cellulite exists can actually make it worse. You see, cellulite (which is basically fat cells that have detached from where they should be) is not actually removed through liposuction. Suctioning the fat around it may make the dimpling effect of the remaining cellulite look worse (but not always; your surgeon will advise you about your specific situation). Also be aware that many parts of the lower body are primarily muscle, so you can't remove much fat from these areas. These include the middle of the buttocks area and the back of the calf.

Before   *After*

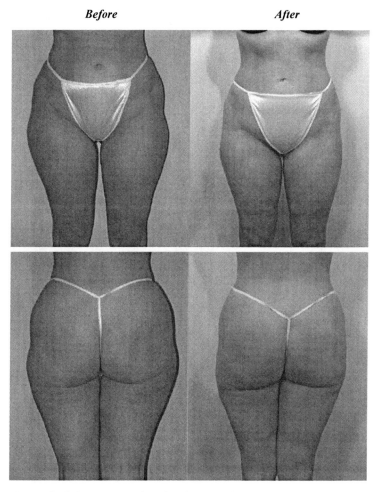

Outer thigh liposuction, female, shown in front view and back view.
(Photos courtesy of Dr. Vince Zubowicz, Atlanta, GA)

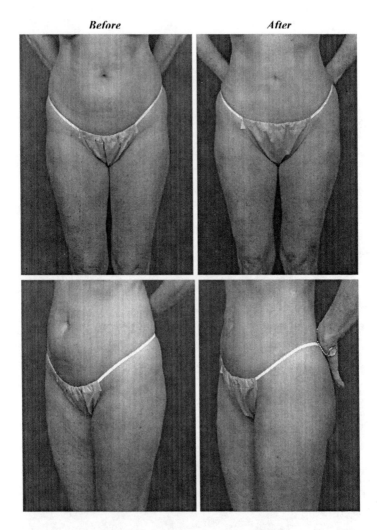

Abdominal liposuction, female, shown in front view and side view.

(Photos courtesy of Dr. Diane Alexander, Atlanta, GA)

How is it done?

Liposuction is usually done on an outpatient basis in the doctor's office operating room or outpatient surgery center, or in a hospital outpatient operating room. But be sure it's an accredited facility! It's still surgery, and some states even limit which liposuction procedures can be done on an outpatient basis. Overnight stay in a hospital is rare. In most lipo, very little blood loss occurs, so there is rarely need for a transfusion. Anesthesia used is either twilight or general. If liposuction is being done in conjunction with an implant, tummy tuck, facelift, or other procedure, everything will typically be done during the same operation.

Depending on the area, surgery itself usually takes about 45 minutes for each section treated. Average overall time for lipoplasty is 45 minutes to 2 hours. You should plan to take four to seven days off work for the first phase of recovery.

How should I prepare?

For the full run-down on preparation, see the previous chapter, of course!

I suggest you buy at least two lipo garments—one black and one beige to go under anything you'll want to wear. "We used to tape everything," Dr. Wells recalls. "We spent a lot of time taping and labeling, and we spent a lot of time pulling it off. Now, the garments come in different sizes, and they are like a body shaper. That's made a big difference."

For about a month after liposuction anywhere on the trunk of your body, **loose-fitting clothes** and underwear will be your best friends (depending on how much you swell). Plan your wardrobe accordingly before surgery. Look for these clothes:

- elastic waistbands (loose or well-padded ones, with fabric covering the elastic, that don't make an indentation—even when it comes to underwear)

- draw-string waist, and (for women) loose dresses with no waist; elastic that makes indentations actually dams up the swelling, making it harder for the swelling to disperse and subside

When you're ready to go back to work, try these:

- waistless dresses

- long jackets

- non-formfitting suits

These are all great for a professional look, while disguising the compression garments you'll be wearing underneath.

Men, you may want to try the following:

- hang on to those suits that begin to get too big as you lose weight, so you can wear them again during this period

- you may also actually go down a shirt neck size after neck liposuction

When all the swelling has gone down and you no longer need the loose-fitting clothes, you may find that you'll need to have your regular clothes taken in—or go get a new wardrobe! While this is a *good* thing, you'll need to keep it in mind when preparing for expenses related to your surgery.

Most people can **return to work within a few days**, depending on how much of the body has been affected and the amount of swelling that occurs. The more areas of the body you have done, the more trauma you will have, and the more time you will need to recover. Of course, it's important to consider what you do in your job. If it involves heavy lifting or other physically demanding labor, you may need to wait longer.

You need to avoid direct exposure to the sun of the treated areas until all bruising has disappeared (usually in two to four weeks), so **don't plan to recover on the beach**!

You'll need to replenish your electrolytes after the dehydrating experience of this surgery. **Stock up on drinks and juices** available at health food stores. Drink lots of water. Sports drinks are good, but they often have too much sodium. Always watch your sodium intake, as it can increase swelling.

You may have drainage from your incisions. In the case of face or chin liposuction, **protect your pillow** with some type of liner, such as a plastic bag under the pillowcase. You'll also need to sleep with your head elevated, so have plenty of pillows ready on your bed for when you get home.

After liposuction of the upper or lower body, **protect your mattress** with some type of bed liner such as dry-cleaning bags, large trash bags, or even a shower curtain under the sheet. A thick towel also can work. You can also see if your drugstore carries the absorbent blue bed liners used by hospitals.

How will I look and feel after surgery?

Don't expect instant gratification. Liposuction can produce quite a bit of swelling and bruising. Remember this as you first see yourself after surgery because you'll look worse than when you went in! Liposuction produces trauma to body tissue, and you will look much worse before you can start looking better. The suctioned areas will be swollen and may bruise. Also, you will actually weigh more after surgery for up to a week, thanks to the fluid pumped into your system. So stay off the scale!

The flip side is that the larger the area on which liposuction is performed, the more quickly you will see the results. The results of little bits of sculpting take longer to emerge from the swelling than do larger amounts of fat removal.

When the local anesthesia wears off, you may feel a burning or throbbing sensation in the suctioned area. Your surgeon may prescribe heavy pain medication for the first day and milder pain medication for subsequent days. You may not even need them. Most people complain of soreness after liposuction but rarely any significant pain.

Different areas will have different types of pain. When I had my stomach done, it felt like I had just done 10,000 sit-ups after never having done them before! The thigh and buttocks areas can be quite painful because there is constant pressure in this area, whether you are standing or sitting.

Even though you will have fluids pumped into you during surgery, remember that you are undergoing a sucking procedure, which quickly takes fluids out. This causes dehydration similar to diarrhea or vomiting and can produce headaches and dry mouth. This is why it's important to get electrolytes back into the body with electrolyte-rich beverages that are low in sodium.

What else do I need to know about recovery?

After surgery, the treated area may be taped, then covered with a **snug elastic dressing**, to control swelling and encourage the skin to shrink back against the underlying tissue. If you are taped, the tape is removed after a few days, and stitches will be removed after seven to ten days. If there is any tape remaining, you will need to remove it very carefully, or it will pull your skin off! Carefully pull up a corner, and get warm water and baby oil under the tape, working it to loosen the adhesive as you go. If you use oil in the shower, be really careful—it'll make the bottom of the tub or shower very slippery!

Remember that pressure on healing wounds causes scars to be more uniform, smaller, and stronger. So, keep that in mind when you feel like shedding your wrappings!

You'll continue wearing a **compression garment** for some time. Every doctor is different, with some who don't even believe in using compression garments, but most will want you to wear one for a few weeks. After that, some doctors will have you wear it as much as possible, at least at night, for a month or two. I believe what some doctors recommend, that the longer you wear it, the better.

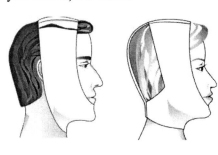

There is a variety of compression garments used for different areas of the body on which liposuction can be performed. These include a face girdle or chin strap for facial liposuction, stockings of various lengths for legs, sleeves for arms, and other types of garments, as seen on this and the next page.

The garment or dressing chosen should provide uniform, steady compression. Doctors will usually only give you one, so during the last consultation with the doctor before your surgery, ask the doctor for another garment so you have a clean one while one is being laundered. You can also purchase additional garments.

135

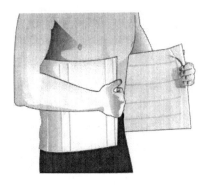
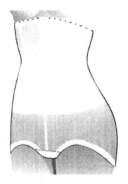

Most doctors will recommend that you **wear the garment at all times for about four weeks**. You'll actually feel better with it on, so it won't seem like a chore. Some doctors ask patients to wear garments for up to 6 months. The older you are, the longer you'll probably need to wear it—our skin becomes less elastic with age (it's hateful, but it's true!).

You'll be able to remove your lipogarment for short periods, like taking a shower, but don't dally in putting it back on—

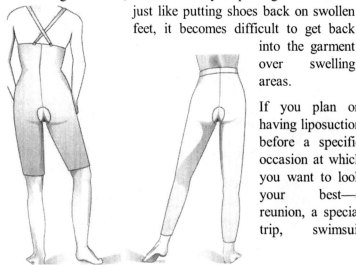

just like putting shoes back on swollen feet, it becomes difficult to get back into the garment over swelling areas.

If you plan on having liposuction before a specific occasion at which you want to look your best—a reunion, a special trip, swimsuit season—keep the recovery time in mind. You don't want to wait until May to have your surgery and still be wearing your lipogarment in June when everyone else is at the beach.

Compression garments may take a little getting used to but can get quite comfortable. One client of mine told me that her lower body stocking felt much like the exercise leggings she was used to wearing when working out, except that it has a large cutout section that allows you go to the bathroom without removing the garment. Then she told me how getting comfortable wearing it actually worked against her one day (this is a funny story, and she laughs about it now, too!):

> She was sitting at home, in her compression "leggings" and a t-shirt, and decided she wanted to get some groceries. She drove to the market down the street. As she browsed the aisles for a healthy snack, she felt a breeze on her bottom. She suddenly realized that she had forgotten to put sweatpants on over her compression garment—and that her bum was hanging out for all to see! She sidled along the wall to the door, quickly got in her car and drove home, hoping no one had noticed! She never did get her snack that day...

The most uncomfortable areas after liposuction tend to be the **thighs, buttocks, and hips,** as there is pressure on them whether you're standing, sitting, or lying down. Some doctors may recommend **massage or ultrasound** treatment of the suctioned areas to decrease swelling and speed recovery. These and other post-

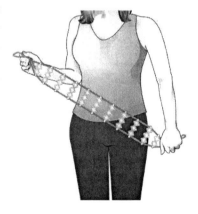

operative therapies are not proven in any clear way to actually benefit healing, but they also don't do any harm. You can massage yourself, too, using a variety of household items such as a rolling pin, paint roller, wooden ball massagers—whatever works for you. After liposuction on my hips, I would watch TV while massaging myself with a lint roller! Whether you choose self-massage or go to a professional, make sure to ask your doctor when it is safe to begin massage.

When liposuction is done on the **lower body**, surgeons advocate a **speedy return to normal activity and work**. Sitting still with your feet hanging down allows fluid to collect, increasing the chances of clot formation. You can begin walking as soon as you wake up from anesthesia. This is limited somewhat after treatment of the legs because too much standing or walking can increase swelling. In any case, total bed rest is *not* necessary or advised, but you should avoid strenuous activities for two to four weeks.

Although **no special diet** is required, results are enhanced by a well-balanced diet and an effort not to overeat. Vitamin C, iron, and zinc supplements may be recommended; always talk to your doctor about anything you may want to take.

"The introduction of some of the herbal products has made a difference in terms of how people deal with bruising," Dr. Wells adds. "Many surgeons like the use of bromelain[4] or arnica[5] products to help with that."

---

4 **bromelain:** an enzyme found in pineapples that breaks down other proteins, such as collagen and muscle fiber, and has anti-inflammatory properties

5 **arnica:** a perennial herb of the genus *Arnica*; a tincture of dried flowers applied to reduce pain and inflammation of bruises and sprains

Liposuction recovery times

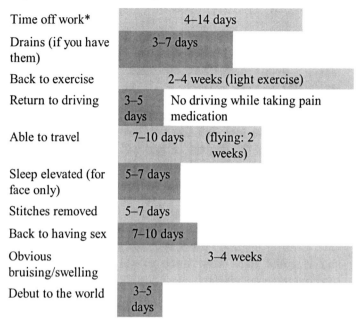

Time off work*	4–14 days
Drains (if you have them)	3–7 days
Back to exercise	2–4 weeks (light exercise)
Return to driving	3–5 days No driving while taking pain medication
Able to travel	7–10 days (flying: 2 weeks)
Sleep elevated (for face only)	5–7 days
Stitches removed	5–7 days
Back to having sex	7–10 days
Obvious bruising/swelling	3–4 weeks
Debut to the world	3–5 days

*Depending on how much is done.

The chart above represents typical healing times. Remember, you will discuss your specific situation with your doctor and listen to what he recommends for you.

It's all part of healing, so don't freak out if...

• ...you experience excessive bruising. This is normal for some people. Most bruises dissipate by the end of two weeks. Though rare, there are some people who stay bruised for up to six weeks.

• ...you experience a burning sensation. After abdominal liposuction, you may feel like you have just done about 10,000 sit-ups! Getting out of bed will be one the more difficult things to do. I'll give you some tips on making it easier on yourself in the chapter on recovery.

• ...the suctioned area looks larger than before the procedure. This is due to swelling as well as fluids that have been injected into the area. Each person is different and it could take from three to six months for the swelling to completely subside.

• ...you experience numbness in the area. This is only temporary and should subside within one year (sometimes people will have small spots that are permanently numb).

• ...the site itches. Don't scratch! Try applying a cold pack to soothe the skin. You may also want to take an oral antihistamine, or use a topical anti-itch medication like spray Benadryl—but remember to ask your doctor before using any medication.

• ...the area becomes hard and lumpy. This is a normal phase of the healing process, and it will soften again.

• ...you have strange sensations during healing. It may feel like warm liquid is running down your skin, or like something is crawling under your skin. Some people even experience what feels like small electric shocks. These are all good signs that healing is taking place!

- ...excessive fluid leaks from your incisions. This is due to the fluid that was injected during the procedure. Mini pads over the incision areas work well for absorption—I know this sounds strange, but it WORKS! Have a supply on hand just in case. Be sure to get mini pads and *not* panty liners—they don't work. If you're a man, you might want to have a female help you with the huge selection.

- ...you have abdominal liposuction and your genital area swells, bruises, and feels numb. This occurs in both sexes. It will typically subside within a few days. (I was shocked after having liposuction on my stomach...I looked down and thought I had an eggplant growing between my legs!)

- ...one side looks more swollen than the other. This asymmetry will right itself as you heal.

- ...if you weigh more right after surgery than you did before you went in. You've had lots of fluids pumped in.

What are the possible risks?

Every operation has risks. Most happen very rarely, but doctors and other medical staff must make you aware of them all...beside, you should want to know about them. There are ways to avoid many risks, and this is one of the reasons you're reading this book!

Depending on how much fat is removed, **sagging skin** can develop in the liposuctioned area. For example, if fat is suctioned from the jowls, and the skin then sags, a facelift can be performed to tighten that skin. If fat is suctioned from the abdomen, and the skin then sags, a tummy tuck can tighten the skin (this goes for both sexes).

Asymmetry (one side of the face or body not matching the other) sometimes requires a second procedure. This is most common for the medial thighs.

Although rare, **pigmentation changes** in the treated area may become permanent if exposed to sun. So keep the treated area out of the sun... you can work on that tan later and, when you do, always wear sun block on scars (and all over, for that matter).

There is a small chance (5–15%) of needing **revision** (a second procedure) for loose skin.

Although this seldom happens, there is a slight chance that **incision scars** may not heal well. This can happen when incisions are made in discreet areas, where the body bends most. Depending on how well you heal, there is also the chance of incision sites becoming thick and scarred. If a scar does not heal to your satisfaction, you can talk to your doctor about scar revision.

Persistent **numbness** at the incision is another rare result.

As with any surgery, there are risks such as **infection** and **blood clots**, though they rarely occur in liposuction performed by a qualified surgeon. To prevent blood clots, be sure to move around as much as your doctor recommends.

There's an *extremely* slight risk of **perforation** of the throat or mouth (in facial liposuction) or intestines (in abdominal liposuction) by the cannula—but it would take a tremendously unqualified surgeon to have that happen!

How much does it cost?

Surgeons' fees for liposuction range from $1,800 to $4,000, depending on the area of the body and the type of procedure used. In 2006, the national average paid for liposuction surgical fees was about $2,900.[6]

Liposuction of the chin or jowls is among the least expensive procedures. If your surgeon recommends liposuction in conjunction with other facial or neck surgery, the liposuction will be included in the total price. Basically, you should count on at least $1,800 for each area that will be liposuctioned.

---

[6]Statistics are from the America Society for Aesthetic Plastic Surgery.

"It's been a week ... why don't I look normal?"

Surgery is, by definition, an invasive technique. When the body is manipulated surgically, it involves cutting, repositioning, putting something in, or taking something out. Mostly, the body doesn't like that being done to it! When you have liposuction, your body undergoes a certain amount of trauma. It's been invaded, and it takes time for the body to get over the attack.

That "getting over it" is what we'll talk about in this chapter.

General recovery and healing

There is a wide variety of recovery periods and phases, based on what you've had done, how well prepared you were, and how appropriate a candidate you are (what body type you have, your age, possible medical conditions, and so on).

- The first and most important thing to remember is that— given time, good nourishment, and proper care—**the body does best at healing itself**. Be patient, be kind, and do what your doctor tells you!

- The second important thing to remember is that **the healing process is just that—a process**. It takes the time it takes. Think about accidental cuts you've had and how long they took to heal. Some surgical procedures involve more trauma to the body than others and, therefore, take more healing time than others. Different people also take different amounts of time to heal.

- The third important point is that your mind will tell you it's ready to "go"—but your body will tell you what you *really* need. **Listen to your body!** When you ignore it and rush it, you put yourself at risk for complications and you interfere with the final results taking shape. The most excellent results of cosmetic procedures happen in recovery, not surgery.

Stitches

Liposuction involves stitches (also known as sutures) or staples (very rarely used) to close the cannula entry sites. Stitches are minimal with liposuction, but for the stitches you do have, keep the following in mind.

- When recovering from liposuction, keep your hands away from the surgical wounds to avoid bacterial contamination.

- Do not let anyone other than the doctor or nurses touch the sutures, and they should only do so while wearing surgical gloves.

- Your doctor will give you instructions for changing the bandages and for showering or sponge bathing (**NO TUB BATHS, HOT TUBS, or SWIMMING POOLS—or lakes, ponds, or oceans!**—are allowed until all the stitches are removed, and then only with the doctor's permission).

- Do not scratch the sutured area or pull sutures that seem to be loose.

- Be careful when you're drying off with a towel—pat dry, don't rub—as a stitch may get caught in the towel fibers.

- Avoid the use of any lotions, creams, oils, cosmetics, medications, or cleaning solutions on or near the wound unless you have your doctor's approval or instructions to do so.

- If instructed to clean your incisions, always wash your hands with anti-bacterial soap before doing so.

- Until incision sites heal, you may have some fluid leakage after surgery, so cover your bedding for the first couple days.

Follow-up visits to the surgeon

Following surgery, you will have follow-up visits with your surgeon. These are done to make sure there are no problems with healing and to do follow-ups like removal of drains and stitches. The follow-up visit schedule will vary depending on the type of liposuction you had and how involved it was.

Your follow-up schedule might include a three-day visit, a one-week visit, a two-week visit, a one-month visit, a three-month visit (which is when the first "after" photos are usually taken), a six-month visit, and a one-year visit. However, if you have had significant liposuction or certain facial procedures, there may be daily contact with the doctor or the doctor's office for the first few days after the procedure.

Follow-up appointments are usually included in the price you pay the doctor for the operation. But be sure to inquire whether follow-up appointments are included in the surgical fee or are additional.

Have your doctor's number and pharmacy number readily available and **call your doctor if you have any of the following:**

- excessive pain (On a scale of 1 to 10, if your pain is anything above a 6, contact the doctor.)

- excessive bleeding

- flu-like symptoms

- area of procedure that is very red and hot to the touch

- oozing yellow fluid from incision

- extreme discomfort

- rash or itching

- excessive vomiting

- nausea from pain pills (You may need different medicine.)

- extreme asymmetry (For example, one liposuctioned thigh is twice as large as the other; one side of your face is twice as swollen.)

- excessive swelling of the feet

It's better to be safe than sorry! Keep in mind that doctors' offices have business hours, too, and try not to wait until 4:55 p.m. on Friday afternoon to call about something! If you have an emergency, by all means have the doctor paged.

How long will recovery take?

Don't base your recovery time on anyone else's. Some people have surgery and are black and blue for three weeks, as I always am (just call me the bruise queen), while others barely have a bruise after surgery. It has very little to do with the doctor or the technique used. It has more to do with your body's tolerance for trauma.

While your recovery time will be individual to you, there are some rules of thumb that can help you plan. The chart on page 139 provides some typical recovery times for liposuction, but your doctor will provide more specific guidelines for your particular procedure.

Black and blue and puffy all over

Swelling and bruising from surgery can last anywhere from a few days to over a month. Remember that these stages are a normal part of healing.

Bruising

It's inevitable, even though bruising affects some people more than others. Once in a blue moon, I'll have the "miracle client" who doesn't bruise. I've also heard of bruises lasting six months. Just remember that a bruise is nothing more than blood trapped under the skin.

The good news is that bruises on the face and neck can be covered up by make-up, and clothes cover bruising on the rest of the body. Keep in mind that discoloration (like everything else) is more apparent to you than to others.

Like everything, bruises are affected by gravity and often migrate. Bruises "shift south" as healing progresses. As an example, if you've had your hips liposuctioned, don't be surprised if the bruising moves to your upper thighs.

The typical life cycle of a bruise is about two weeks. A quick healer may lose bruises in four days, an average healer in seven to ten days, and a slow healer may have traces left after three weeks. Bruises often appear their worst on the third or fourth day, when they "peak." At that point, you can take comfort in the fact that they won't get worse! Typical bruise color stages include brown, red, blue, green, and yellow. There is a form of bruise that turns yellow right away (yes, it lasts just as long as the black and blue kind!).

If your bruising keeps getting worse after the fourth day, **notify your doctor**. A bruise that appears red and feels hot may be a sign of hematoma[7] and/or infection.

To **help prevent bruising**, you'd be wise to stay away from drugs, supplements, and herbs that can affect how your blood clots and thereby cause bruising or make it worse. For example, aspirin (acetylsalicylic acid) can increase bleeding and swelling because it interferes with the normal clotting ability of blood platelets. Some other medications, such as **ibuprofen**, **vitamin E**, and **blood-thinning drugs** can also lead to increased bleeding. The list below is compiled from a number of sources, including doctors' recommendations and information from the Journal of the American Medical Association (JAMA).

aspirin	marine fatty acids	garlic
ibuprofen, Motrin, Advil	omega-3 fish oil supplements	ginkgo
Naproxen, Aleve	chondroitin	ginseng
Vitamin E	feverfew	

To be safe, if you take any of these on a regular basis, stop taking it a week or two before you have your liposuction. If you're taking aspirin (or anything else) as directed by a physician, talk to your doctor about risks of both continuing and stopping your regimen.

If you bruise very easily or your bruises last a long time, talk to your surgeon about bruise preventions. The following ingredients are commonly used to lessen bruising:

---

7 **hematoma:** localized bleeding or blood clot under the skin

- Arnica[8], though classified as a potentially dangerous herb by the FDA, is safely available in some mixtures from reputable homeopathic companies to help prevent bruising (topical or oral; check the Internet or a local health food store).

- Fresh pineapple has an enzyme that helps bring down bruising and swelling.

- Vitamin K is sometimes prescribed; ask your doctor (some doctors also recommend Vitamin C).

Typically, local anesthesia, as well as the wetting solution that is injected, contains an agent (epinephrine[9]) that also helps prevent bruising.

Swelling

Swelling is another aftermath of surgery that no one can avoid. It's a natural stage of wounds healing. Again, some people swell more than others, and for longer periods. You can pretty easily cover up swelling anywhere on the body with clothing. Unfortunately, it's harder to hide facial swelling. Again, remember that it'll be more noticeable to you than to anyone else—it's amazing how unobservant people are … unless it's your mother!

Swelling is usually at its worst for about a week following liposuction. Depending on what you've had done, some swelling can remain for several weeks afterward.

To help keep swelling down:

---

8 **arnica:** see page 113

9 **epinephrine:** adrenaline

- Drink as much liquid as possible—water, juice, caffeine-free tea (caffeine is a diuretic, so stay away from that, and be careful of certain herb teas—ask your doctor about which teas are OK). Stay away from drinks with sodium such as soda and some sports drinks; to find out sodium contents, read the labels!

- Wear your compression garment. The constant and equal pressure it applies to the area is very effective in reducing swelling.

- After lipo of the face and/or neck, keep your head above your heart. Sleeping in almost a sitting position is best.

- Some sources say that swelling may be caused or made worse by taking **Ephedra (ma huang)**, **goldenseal**, and—of all things—**licorice**.

One complication to watch for is seroma[10], which can look like normal swelling at first. Seromas are common after some liposuction, tummy tucks, and some facelifts. You can tell a seroma from normal swelling because it's fluidy. If you suspect a seroma, you should call your doctor. Seromas need to be aspirated[11]—in some cases, several times—but they usually don't hurt and are not an emergency.

---

10 **seroma:** liquid under the skin; a mass or swelling caused by the localized accumulation of serum within a tissue or organ

11 **aspiration:** removal of fluid through a needle

The thing about scars

Where you're cut, you're gonna have a scar!

Whenever an incision is made, damage is done to skin, tissue, blood vessels, and nerves. Surgeons who perform liposuction are experts in closing incisions so that scars heal as inconspicuously as possible. However, all incisions will produce some scarring. No scar is absolutely invisible, although many scars will become less noticeable with time.

At first, a scar will appear red and hard. This is normal and may last three to six months. After that, it will start to soften. If it doesn't soften within a time limit determined by you and your surgeon, a steroid shot can soften the scar. Some doctors believe in doing this early on, while others use it as a last resort if natural healing is not producing the desired result.

After several months, scars may fade to a fine line. Sometimes scars are larger and thicker than you might like or expect. Make-up and hair can usually cover scars from liposuction of the face and neck, and of course, clothing normally hides scars on the body. The most obvious surgical scars are left after operations in areas where there are no natural skin folds to hide them. For example, there is no natural fold to hide the incision for a tummy tuck or a breast reduction or liposuction of the back.

Your doctor may advise that you use an over-the-counter antibacterial lotion on your surgical wound. After the stitches are removed, some people use things such as vitamin-enriched skin lotions, aloe vera, and even vitamin E oil to coat the scar. These may aid in healing and result in a less noticeable scar. Be aware that oil applied to a wound may cause infection. Another option is using a silicone strip, which adheres to the skin and helps the scar heal evenly. Ask your doctor before applying any lotion, cream, or other product to your surgical wound.

There are some interesting facts about scars:

- **Mirror-image scars** (scars from incisions in identical places on both sides of the face or body) never heal in the same way. They take on different sizes and shapes and take different amounts of time to heal. One side inevitably will look better than the other.

- As long as a scar is **red or pink, it is still healing**. The healing process—which should eventually yield a scar that is thin and flat—can take a couple of months (some facial scars can heal that fast, as the face is exposed to air and has so many blood vessels) to more than a year (scars hidden in skin folds, which don't get air or light and may bend and stretch constantly, can take much longer).

- Make-up can easily **disguise most scars** on the face. I have seen both women and men do a wonderful job of hiding surgical scars without it looking as though they are "wearing make-up."

Ideally, a scar should almost blend with your skin color. For Caucasians, well-healed scars become thin and white; for people with darker skin, scars should be skin-tone or a little darker.

If a scar does not heal the way you were hoping it would, it can usually be fixed. This is called a **scar revision**. The first thing to find out is how long you need to wait before you and your doctor can see whether natural healing will take the scar to the stage where you'll be satisfied. Keep in mind that this is additional procedure, and plan for another recovery period.

Keeping tabs on your progress

People never heal as fast as they think they should. No one wants to hear or believe this (not even me!), but the healing process can take up to a year. That's one full year.

A great way to see the progression of your healing is to have someone photograph the area once every three to four days for the first month. (You can use a tripod and self-timer if you don't want someone else taking the photos.) Then, take a photo once every two weeks for the next two months. The pictures should all be taken in the same location, with the same lighting and at the same distance for accurate comparison. Unlike looking in the mirror every day, this photo journal gives you a great overview of how far your healing has come. Remember, Rome wasn't built in a day. Have **patience** with the process. It will happen.

Giving your body what it needs

Your doctor should provide you with instructions as to when you can begin **normal hygiene** such as bathing, showering, shaving, washing your hair, and wearing make-up. Unless you are given other instructions, do not put any creams or ointments on your stitches.

You will also be instructed as to when you can gradually become active again with workout activities and **daily routines**. Looking after your emotional well-being and keeping stress levels down are also important factors in your recovery.

If you have **pets**, it is probably a good idea not to have them around for a few days. I say this because you will need plenty of rest and will not be able to care for your pets for the first few days. Also, make sure you vacuum and dust thoroughly wherever you are going to be recovering in order to remove as much fur and dust as possible.

Getting a **good night's sleep** is imperative after any surgical procedure (see the *Sleep* section, beginning on page 110). Your body needs rest and time to heal. Any steps you take to ensure proper rest will be well worth the effort. I always suggest getting things ready at home to make it easier (see *Preparing your home*, starting on page 104, for tips).

Return to having sex

After many procedures, you won't feel very romantic. With some, you should avoid having sex for a while anyway. When you are able to and feel comfortable with returning to sex, you may need to get a little creative to avoid pain or interference with your healing. You don't want to stretch an incision site or otherwise harm yourself!

Some creative sexual positions are featured in books about the Kama Sutra, available in almost any bookstore and through the Internet.

Getting in and out of bed

This may be a challenge at first, too. The most important thing is to **TAKE IT SLOW**! If you move too fast getting out of bed, you have a good chance of passing out—no matter what procedure you've had.

After lipo of the face: You're already in a seated position. Shift so that you can swing your legs over the side of the bed, then put your feet firmly on the floor. Sit still in this position for 30 seconds. Then stand up **S-L-O-W-L-Y**, and stand there for 30 seconds (take a couple of deep breaths to get oxygen flowing through your body) before you begin walking. If you get dizzy, you want to make sure that the bed is still behind you! And remember, no bending over to put on slippers or socks!

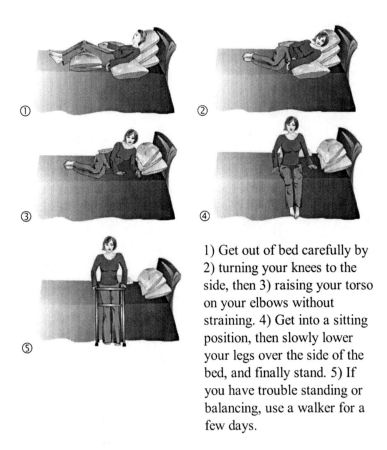

1) Get out of bed carefully by 2) turning your knees to the side, then 3) raising your torso on your elbows without straining. 4) Get into a sitting position, then slowly lower your legs over the side of the bed, and finally stand. 5) If you have trouble standing or balancing, use a walker for a few days.

After liposuction of the tummy, or a tummy tuck: The last thing you want to do is use your abdominal muscles. To avoid getting pinched or poked by someone helping you get up, use a big towel for leverage (see the illustration). There are two ways to get out of bed—one is to roll over on your side (yes, this will hurt, too), keep yourself in a fetal position, then push yourself up with your arms. From this position, you slowly lower your

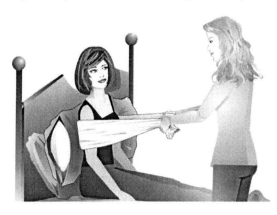

feet to the floor. If your bed is high, you might want to have some sort of stable step beside it so you don't have to stretch your legs so far.

The second way is to have a rope tied underneath the bottom of the bed that you can use to pull yourself up (there are ready-made devices available for this purpose; use the Internet or call a local medical supply company).

Showering and bathing

Here are some tips for when your physician gives you permission to take a **bath or shower**:

- No matter what procedure you've had done, I strongly recommend you have someone stand close by the first three showers you take. You may get light-headed.

- You may want to consider sitting in the shower. I highly recommend this. You can use an ordinary plastic lawn chair or a shower chair from a medical supply store, catalog, or some drug stores.

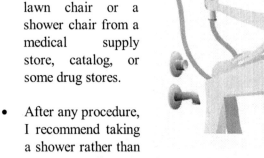

- After any procedure, I recommend taking a shower rather than sitting in a tub. It's easier, and the less you go up and down (sitting to standing), the better. In addition, sitting in water (bathtub, hot tub, Jacuzzi, and so on) is not advisable, as water is full of bacteria and can potentially cause a nasty infection even with the smallest incision.

- Keep the water warm, but not hot, as this could cause further bruising. Make sure the showerhead is set to a gentle spray—no pulsating massages for a while. If you have one, it is ideal to use a hand-held shower and keep the spray from beating directly onto sensitive areas. (And if you've always wanted a hand-held shower, here's a great excuse to get it! They're easy to install—if I can do it, anybody can!)

After lipo of the face:

- After **cheek or chin implants**, or **liposuction of the face or neck**, you can shower as you normally would.

After surgery anywhere on the body:

- If your doctor has given you permission to shower and you still have sutures, be careful you don't catch them with anything (a ring, the washcloth, a sponge).

- After **liposuction**, I suggest getting in the shower with your compression garment on. Wash everything around the garment (hair, face, limbs). Then remove the garment very slowly. Many people get very lightheaded removing their garment for the first time, so have someone standing by. If this happens, immediately lie down on the floor and elevate your legs.

  Wash the garment using shampoo or body wash and rinse it. Wrap it in a towel to soak up excess water, then hang it on the side of the tub or hand it to the person standing by. Wash your body using a light circular motion to get the circulation going. Get out and pat yourself dry carefully. Apply baby powder (preferably one that has corn starch in it) to the area that'll be covered by the garment. This helps the garment slide on easier. Quickly put on a fresh, dry garment—the longer you wait, the more you'll swell, and it'll be harder to get the garment on again. So don't dilly-dally!

Eating properly

You may not feel a whole lot like **eating** for a while. The trauma to your body, plus the medications you'll be taking, may take away much of your appetite. Food may also taste different to you, depending on the medication you're taking. However, it's very important to eat healthy foods to speed healing.

- Remember to **plan ahead** and think about how much food you'll need to have on hand before you're able to go out and shop for more. This will depend on the type of procedure you're having and its approximate recovery time.

- Be sure to have food and beverages that are **low in sodium and salt**, so as not to cause even more swelling. Also stay away from soft drinks, spicy foods, frozen dinners, canned foods, alcohol, and so on. Read labels, and stock up on as much fresh and natural food as possible.

- There's nothing worse than not feeling hungry and having to eat. But you have to put healthy food in your body! If you just can't face food, be sure to at least have a **protein drink or high-protein snack**. You need to get into a regular routine of eating balanced meals as soon as possible.

- Remember that you **can't take certain medications on an empty stomach**. Be sure to read thoroughly the instructions on each drug, as some say to take with food and some an hour or two after eating.

Back on your feet

I've repeated this many times, but it bears saying again—you can't rush the healing process. Remember that if you do, the damage you cause may very easily take longer to deal with than if you had let healing run its course in the first place.

> A former client came to see me about breast augmentation. She decided on implants below the muscle, a technique that causes a little more trauma to the body than implants above the muscle.
>
> After her operation, she had rounded the corner of the intense part of healing—the first week or so. On the tenth day, she felt pretty good, and she thought she was ready to go back to doing some things around the house.
>
> An avid gardener, she went out and began playing in her garden. It happened to need fertilizing, so what does she do? She lifts a 40-pound bag of fertilizer!
>
> Later that night, she called me, asking why she might be in severe pain at this stage of her recovery. It took me a while to get it out of her. I had to mentally walk her through her day, until we came upon the fact that she had done heavy lifting.
>
> We called her doctor and went in the next day for him to check if everything was all right. It turned out she was fine. She was lucky. The lifting could have caused a hematoma[12], or she may have had to have more surgery.

---

12 **hematoma:** see page 115

The moral of that story is: Even if your head tells you that you're fine and can do more, listen to your doctor and wait for him to tell you when it's OK to do things as you recover.

Some activities, such as going for walks, may help you recover faster. Find out what you can and cannot do during recovery and how the surgical wound will affect your mobility. Various movements may have to be avoided so there will be no strain to the incisions or the surgical wound.

On page 139, you will find a chart that shows typical waiting times for getting back into certain activities. Use it as a guide, but remember to ask your surgeon how long you specifically should wait.

Prepare to heal well:
Your Post-Surgical Checklist

Some tips to make your recovery as painless as possible:

☐ Make sure you take a proper amount of **time off from work**. Consult with your doctor and take all the time that he recommends…or even a little more. Check the chart on page 139 for standard recovery times (but remember that everyone heals differently).

☐ Have a list of **restaurants that deliver** to your area. Also, have **meals prepared and ready** for your recovery at home. Keep away from salty or spicy foods. Check sodium content in canned foods and soft drinks. Sodium will make you swell.

☐ Have all **prescriptions filled prior to surgery**. It is a good idea to keep a written record of when you take what amount to avoid losing track of appropriate dosages and times. A pill box with days and times on the compartments will help.

☐ Have your bed freshly made and your **room prepared** for your arrival after surgery, with extra pillows for propping up.

☐ Stock up on **videos to watch and books to read,** or have other activities ready for the recovery period.

☐ **Follow your doctor's post-op instructions**.

☐ **Don't do anything your doctor tells you not to do**. If, for some reason, you forget and do something you weren't supposed to do, be honest with your doctor and tell him. This is very important.

☐ If your doctor gives you a sleeping pill to take the night before your surgery, take it. It is very important to get a **full eight hours of sleep before your operation**.

☐ Have **straws to drink with** or a sippy cup.

☐ Have your doctor's and pharmacy's **telephone numbers close at hand**. Make sure you have a **friend or family member you can rely on** in case of an emergency.

☐ Find a **24-hour drug store** close to your home and/or one that delivers.

☐ Have **anti-bacterial soap** on hand.

☐ Make sure you have two **night lights** (one as back-up) or some form of low wattage light in the bedroom and the bathroom to avoid any accidents in the dark.

☐ Make arrangements to have **reliable transportation** home and **reliable help at home** for at least the first day or two (longer after some procedures).

☐ Have a **bell to ring or a baby monitor** so you don't need to shout for assistance.

☐ Make sure that your **air conditioner** is running in hot weather, or that the house is **warm in the winter**.

ON THE RIDE HOME, THE PERSON DRIVING YOU SHOULD BRING:

☐ A **wet washcloth** placed in a zip-locked bag with ice cubes. This is in case of nausea.

☐ A **plastic bag or bowl** in case of vomiting.

☐ A **towel**.

☐ A **sunshade** to place on the passenger side window to block the sun and for privacy.

164

Medical Boards

In this section, you will find information about pertinent boards of the American Board of Medical Specialties (ABMS) and how each one certifies doctors. There are 24 medical boards at this writing, but the only ones listed here are those you will want to know about when having cosmetic surgery.

A physician's board certification is valid for 10 years. In order to remain board-certified, the physician must pass a re-certification test every 10 years.

To find out more about medical boards, visit the ABMS Web site at **www.abms.org**. On the site, you can search for whether a physician is certified by one of these boards by completing a search free of charge (**www.abms.org/newsearch.asp**), or you can call the ABMS certification line at 1-800-776-2378.

American Board of Anesthesiology

Requirements for Board Certification

Candidate shall be capable of performing independently the entire scope of anesthesiology practice and must:

- Have graduated from medical school or from a school of osteopathy in the U.S., Canada or foreign medical school (in which case the graduate must have a certificate from the Educational Commission for Foreign Medical Graduates (ECFMG)

- Hold a permanent, unconditional, unrestricted and unexpired license to practice medicine in the U.S. or Canada

- Have satisfactorily completed the training requirement before the examination date. (training must begin after applicant receives a medical degree, in a residency program approved by the ABA)

- Have fulfilled requirements of the Continuum of Education in

Anesthesiology, which include:

- Satisfactory completion of <u>1 year of Clinical Base training</u> and <u>3 years of Clinical Anesthesia Training</u> by August 31 of the year in which the written Board examination is given.

- Have on file with the American Board of Anesthesiology a <u>Certificate of Clinical Competence</u> with an overall satisfactory rating covering the final six-month period of Clinical Anesthesia training in each anesthesiology residency program.

- Have on file with the Board evaluations of various aspects of his/her current practice of anesthesiology.

- Have satisfied all examination requirements (oral and written) of the Board.

- Have a moral, ethical and professional standing satisfactory to the ABA

You can mail a request for board status verification along with a $10.00 check to:

American Board of Anesthesiology
4101 Lake Boone Trail, Suite 510
Raleigh, NC 27607-7506
(919)881-2570; Web site: http://www.abanes.org

Mailed request must include physician's name and ABA identification number (made up of physician's SSN & birth date).

American Board of Dermatology

If you want to have a dermatologist do a cosmetic procedure, you will want to make sure he is certified by this board. For the most part, doctors of dermatology can perform the following cosmetic procedures:

- Chemical peel
- Dermabrasian
- Hair restoration
- Injectables (such as Botox and collagen)
- Laser resurfacing
- Liposuction
- Spider and varicose veins
- Tattoo removal
- and other skin-related procedures.

Requirements for Board Certification

Candidate shall be capable of performing independently the entire scope of dermatology practice and must:

- Have graduated from a medical school in the U.S., Canada or foreign medical school with ECFMG certification.

- Have a currently valid, full and unrestricted license to practice medicine or osteopathy in the U.S. or Canada.

- Have completed 4 years of postgraduate training including:

    - 1 year of residency training (first year after graduation) in internal medicine, general surgery, family practice, obstetrics & gynecology, pediatrics, or emergency medicine.

    - 3 years of full-time training as a resident in a dermatology residency training program in the U.S. or Canada.

- Pass the written and oral board certification examination.

- Have a moral, ethical and professional standing satisfactory to the board.

The American Board of Dermatology
Henry Ford Hospital
One Ford Plaza
Detroit, MI 48202-3450
(517) 332-4800 ; Web site: www.abderm.org

American Board of Ophthalmology

If you want to have an ophthalmologist do a cosmetic procedure, you will want to make sure he is certified by this board. Doctors of ophthalmology can perform cosmetic procedures having to do with the eye (such as upper and lower blepharoplasty) and some do perform browlifts.

Requirements for Board Certification

Candidate shall be capable of performing independently the entire scope of dermatology practice and must:

- Have graduated from medical school or from a school of osteopathy in the U.S., Canada or foreign medical school with ECFMG certification.

- Have a currently valid, full and unrestricted license to practice medicine in the U.S. or Canada

- Have completed 4 to 5 years of postgraduate training including:

  - 1 year of post-graduate training in internal medicine, general surgery, family practice, obstetrics & gynecology, pediatrics, or emergency medicine.

  - 3 to 4 years of full-time training as a resident in an ophthalmology residency training program in the U.S. or Canada

- Pass the written and oral board certification.

- Have a moral, ethical and professional standing satisfactory to the board.

The American Board of Ophthalmology
111 Presidential Blvd., Suite 241
Bala Cynwyd, PA 19004
(610) 664-1175 (To check board status); Web site: www.abop.org

American Board of Otolaryngology

If you want to have an otolaryngologist (ear, nose, throat doctor) do
a cosmetic procedure, you will want to make sure he is certified by
this board. Doctors of otolaryngology can perform the following
cosmetic procedures:

- Blepharoplasty (eyes)
- Brow lift
- Chin and cheek implants
- Ear pinning
- Facelift
- Rhinoplasty (nose job)
- and other procedures of the head and neck.

Requirements for Board Certification

Candidate shall be capable of performing independently the entire
scope of Otolaryngology (head & neck surgery) practice and must:

- Have graduated from a medical school in the U.S. or Canada or
  foreign medical school with ECFMG certification

- Have a currently valid, full and unrestricted license to practice
  medicine or osteopathy in the U.S. or Canada.

- Have completed <u>5 years</u> of postgraduate residency training
  including:
  - 1 year of general surgery training
  - 4 years of residency training in otolaryngology-head and
    neck surgery.

- Have on file with the Board a Verification of Otolaryngology
  Residency Form, signed by the residency program director,
  attesting to satisfactory completion of the training program

- Have on file a Yearly Report Form for each year of training,
  signed by the training director. This form certifies satisfactory

completion of each year of training.

- Have on file with the Board an Operative Experience Report for each year of training. This report contains a log of all the surgical procedures that the resident participated in that year.

- Pass the written and oral board certification examination.

- Have a moral, ethical and professional standing satisfactory to the board.

American Board of Otolaryngology
3050 Post Oak Boulevard, Suite 1700
Houston, Texas 77057
(713) 850-0399 (To check board status)
Web site: www.aboto.org

American Board of Plastic Surgery

As the title of this board implies, surgeons certified in plastic surgery can do it all—procedures of the head and body. However, the vast majority of plastic surgeons do specialize. When you find a board-certified plastic surgeon, you're definitely on the right track. Then you need to ask what portion (if any) of his practice is cosmetic surgery (rather than reconstructive), and then if he has a cosmetic surgery specialty. You wouldn't want to have a facelift done by a plastic surgeon whose only cosmetic surgery specialty if breast augmentation.

Requirements for Board Certification

Candidate shall be capable of performing independently the entire scope of Plastic Surgery practice and must:

- Have graduated from a medical school in the U.S. or Canada or foreign medical school with ECFMG certification

- Have a currently valid, full and unrestricted license to practice medicine or osteopathy in the U.S. or Canada.

- Have completed 5 to 6 years of post-graduate residency training including:

171

- minimum <u>3 years</u> of clinical training in general surgery (Alimentary tract, abdomen and its contents, breast/skin and soft tissue, head & neck, vascular system, endocrine system, surgical oncology, comprehensive management of trauma, complete care of critically ill patients with underlying surgical conditions)

- <u>2 to 3 years</u> of plastic surgery residency training (including experience in both the functional and aesthetic (cosmetic) management of congenital and acquired defects of the head and neck, trunk, and extremities.

- Pass the written and oral board certification examination.

- Have a moral, ethical and professional standing satisfactory to the board.

American Board of Plastic Surgery
Seven Penn Center, Suite 400
1635 Market Street
Philadelphia, PA 19103-2204
(215) 587-9322
Web site: www.abplsurg.org

American Board of Surgery

This board is one that certifies general surgeons. It is included as it may be the certification of the surgeon you choose, but again you will want to make sure he specializes in the procedure you want. The more general a certification, the likely it may be that the surgeon has done a great many of any one type of operation. There are exceptions to every rule, but just be aware of this.

Requirements for Board Certification

Candidate shall be capable of performing independently the entire scope of General Surgery practice and must:

- Have graduated from a medical school in the U.S. or Canada or foreign medical school with ECFMG certification

- Have a currently valid, full and unrestricted license to practice medicine or osteopathy in the U.S. or Canada.

- Have completed a <u>minimum of 5 years</u> of progressive post-graduate surgery training including:

  - <u>3 to 4 years</u> of training devoted to the primary components of surgery (Alimentary tract, abdomen and its contents, breast/skin and soft tissue, head & neck, vascular system, endocrine system, surgical oncology, comprehensive management of trauma, complete care of critically ill patients with underlying surgical conditions)

  - <u>1 to 2 years</u> of training as the Chief Resident in General Surgery. During this time the resident assumes the ultimate clinical responsibilities for patient care under the supervision of the teaching staff.

  - completion of a minimum of <u>500 surgical procedures</u> in 5 years including a minimum of <u>150 procedures</u> in the Chief/Senior year.

- Pass the written and oral board certification examination.

- Have a moral, ethical and professional standing satisfactory to the board.

American Board of Surgery
1617 John F. Kennedy Blvd., Suite 860
Philadelphia, PA 19103-1847
(215) 568-0059
Web site: www.absurgery.org

International Information

Here are resources for obtaining information about having surgery somewhere other than in the United States. These are good places to begin gathering information if you live in or plan to have your procedure in any of these places.

International
ISAPS (International Society of Aesthetic Plastic Surgery): Association that provides a listing for its member physicians all over the world.
    Web site: www.isaps.org

Canada
The Royal College of Physicians and Surgeons of Canada
    Web site: www.royalcollege.ca

Mexico
Asociacion Mexicana de Cirugia Plastica, Estetica y Reconstructiva, A.C. (Mexican Association of Plastic, Aesthetic and Reconstructive Surgery)
    Web site: www.plasticsurgery.org.mx

Europe
European Association of Plastic Surgeons
    Web site: www.euraps.org
British Association of Aesthetic Plastic Surgeons
    Web site: www.baaps.org.uk
French Society of Aesthetic Plastic Surgeons
    Web site: www.sofcep.org

South America
Brazilian Society of Plastic Surgeons
    Web site: www.cirurgiaplastica.org.br

Index

risks · 5, 11, 18, 44, 45, 47, 54, 68, 92, 117, 121, 123, 141, 142, 149

T

teenagers · 103
tests · 82, 117, 118
The Informed Choice · 4, 9, 37, 64
tracking progress · 43
transportation · 20, 96, 116, 164
traveling · 58, 112
tumescent · 119, 122, 123
Tylenol · 110

U

Ultrasound-Assisted Lipoplasty · 123

V

vanity · 27, 28
Vitamin C · 138, 150
Vitamin E · 149, 152
Vitamin K · 150
vomiting · 42, 97, 134, 147, 164

W

weight · 16, 24, 32, 46, 55, 69, 110, 125, 126, 132
work · 21, 23, 97, 125, 132, 138
   time off · 20, 76, 97, 131, 139, 163
   time off · 18

1282015

Made in the USA